The Secret of KI.

End of
INJURY

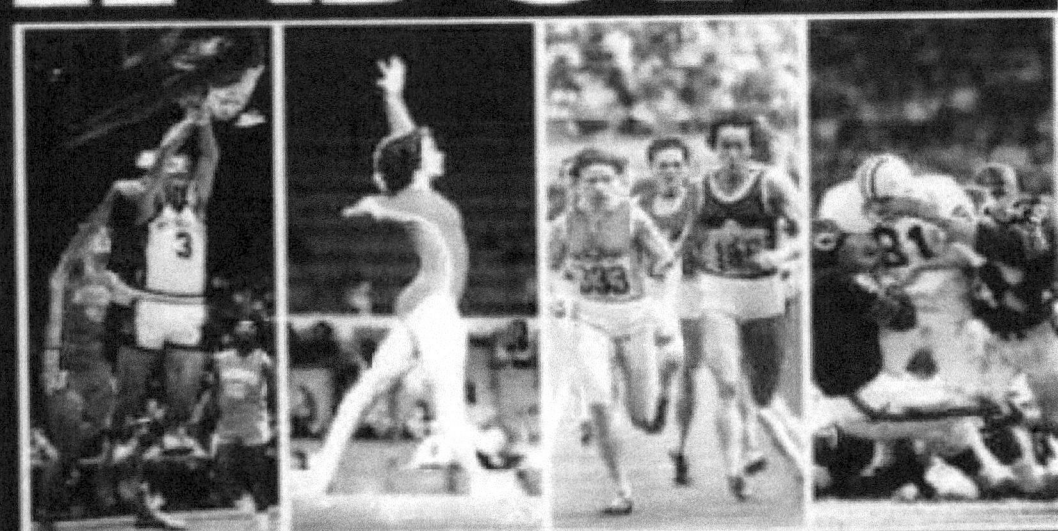

Grandmaster
Ted Gambordella

END OF INJURY

A comprehensive program for the prevention of athletic injuries, improvement of performance, and the development of a positive mental attitude.

By Grandmaster Dr. Ted Gambordella, B.S., M.ED., PhD

INTRODUCTION

I wrote this book because every year there are thousands of needless and unnecessary injuries that occur to professional, collegiate and amateur athletes. It seems that in America, most people do not worry about something until it's too late or till it has already happened. Take for example illness … we spend billions in curing the symptoms of the illness, medicine to stop the drippy nose, ease the pain, relieve the pressure, etc. But we spend very little to prevent the body from becoming ill. Our country spends billions of dollars on medical research to cure illness but only a pittance on research to prevent the illness. The same thing holds true for sports and sport related injuries.

Every year thousands of athletes fall down and break or tear a part of their body. Every year thousands of athletes get hit in the ribs or abdomen and break bones or injure internal organs. Every day someone makes a mistake while playing and finds himself injured perhaps permanently because no coach or no one ever told him how to *PREVENT ATHLETIC INJURIES*. This book does just that, shows easy to follow, proven techniques for the prevention of athletic injuries. Of course this book will not make you a Superman or prevent all injuries. What it will do is to provide you with alternatives. Now you can at least have a chance to roll instead of break, to stretch instead of tear, and to absorb instead of crush your body from most aspects of your sport that can cause injury.

(1). There are only three ways that an injury can occur and there are proven techniques that can help prevent these injuries:

a.   Stretching or flexibility related injuries - pulling or tearing muscles from over stretching the muscles, tendons or ligaments. Solution: a complete stretching program.

b.   Falling down - breaking bones or tearing muscles, joints and the body in general. Solution: proper falling techniques.

c.   Getting hit - contact that breaks bones, injures muscle. Solution: use of Ki (breath, muscle and mind control all used simultaneously).

(2)   A relaxed athlete is able to perform better and less likely to be injured. When you are upset, your body over-reacts and your mind becomes confused so that you are not able to perform at your top level.

(3)   Size and strength can be overcome by the use of balance points and leverage. A child can balance a 400 lb. refrigerator on one corner if he maintains the balance. It took you 2 years to learn to walk and your balance is conditional upon the entire cooperation of your whole body (the eyes, inner ears, toes, arms, hips, etc.). Force can be applied in only one direction and if you learn to utilize the techniques of balance and leverage in this book you can easily maneuver and manipulate a much larger and stronger opponent.

If you will study this book with an open mind, begin to practice the techniques and appreciate the value of the techniques found in it. Your ability to concentrate will greatly improve, your skills will sharpen and your mind becomes stronger. You will have a much greater ability to withstand blows and hits that would injure most people, and you will improve your performance by the use of balance points, concentration and mind control.

Books by Ted Gambordella

SEVEN DAYS TO SELF DEFENSE

THE END OF INJURIES

HOW TO DEVELOP A PERFECT BODY

41 WAYS TO FLATTEN YOUR STOMACH

WEAPONS OF THE STREET

THE COMPLETE BOOK OF KARATE WEAPONS

SECRETS OF STREET FIGHTING

FIGHT FOR YOUR LIFE

THE 100 DEADLIEST KARATE MOVES

TONFA TACTICS

O.M.A. OBSESSIVE MENTAL ATTITUDE

WINNING WITH THE FIRST PUNCH

THE AMAZING SECRETS OF MARTIAL ARTS MASTERS

THE AMAZING SECRETS OF MARTIAL ARTS FITNESS

TIME OUT FOR BULLIES

THE SECRET OF KI

Why the Techniques Found in This Book Will Work

The techniques found in this book come primarily from martial art techniques and many people are prejudiced against martial arts because in America the martial arts do not have the excellent and respected reputation they do in the Orient. The reason due to the fact that many people in America profess themselves to be better than they are and they have too little knowledge and too poor of technique but are going around telling everyone that they are the greatest. Only one person can be the greatest. So they usually find themselves in compromising situations such as breaking their hands trying to break bricks, or getting punched out by a girl. But this does not mean that the techniques and the art form that they have learned are not effective. It only means that they are not effective in using them. A gun will certainly kill you, but first you have to hit the person with the bullet. So martial art techniques are definitely effective but first the person doing them must be able to hit the target with the right technique.

The martial arts are just that, art forms, and as such are beautiful to watch and tend to become a way of life with the true practioners. They are techniques that can be enjoyed and practiced for benefit by anyone, just as any great work of art can be enjoyed by all viewers.

The techniques found in this book do not just come from Karate, which is what many people think of when they hear the words martial arts, but they come from Judo, and Jiu-Jitsu, Kung Fu, Aikido, Kendo, Zen, Yoga, and even psychology and ballet. Techniques that can be applicable to all forms of sports have been utilized in this manual for the mutual benefit of the players and the fans. For no one wants to get hurt or see a player get hurt, and everyone wants maximum performance, a positive attitude and a stronger mind.

Let us examine the facts:

1. There is no better way in the world to learn how to fall without receiving an injury than to practice Judo falling techniques.

2. The most flexible people in the world are ballerinas and karate men. The stretches taken from these two arts will enable you to become as flexible as you wish.

3. There is only one art form in the world that teaches you how to get hit without getting injured: Jiu-Jitsu, and it does not require any magical mystical powers. It is simply breath, muscle and mind control all put together to form a new identity called KI. (Just like the various pieces of metal are all put together and form a new machine called a car.)

4. There is no better form or exercise to develop powers of concentration and mind control than techniques of meditation taken from Zen and Yoga.

5. Aikido is a 2,000 year old art form that enables one to overcome the largest of opponents with the minimal of effort by the use of balance points and leverage.

6. Breathing is both necessary to sustain life and vital in athletic performance, in relaxation and in concentration. If you don't believe me, hold your breath for a week, or try to sleep while breathing 70 times a minute. The best techniques of breath control in the world come from Yoga and its exercises.

7. The most powerful method of striking or hitting another person or thing ever developed comes from Karate techniques of weight shifting and striking. (Ever try to break a brick?)

8. Techniques of one sport can be applied to make other sports more effective.

So please do not find yourself being prejudiced against techniques found in this book before you even try them. They simply are the most effective means man has ever found to do the things described and if you will use them in your sport, you can improve your performance, develop a positive mental attitude and prevent most injuries. Keep an open mind, practice them and apply them in any way you wish. Adapt them to your style and use them at your discretion, but employ them and use them and you and your sport will greatly benefit.

Why the Techniques Found in This Book Will Work

The techniques found in this book come primarily from martial art techniques and many people are prejudiced against martial arts because in America the martial arts do not have the excellent and respected reputation they do in the Orient. The reason due to the fact that many people in America profess themselves to be better than they are and they have too little knowledge and too poor of technique but are going around telling everyone that they are the greatest. Only one person can be the greatest. So they usually find themselves in compromising situations such as breaking their hands trying to break bricks, or getting punched out by a girl. But this does not mean that the techniques and the art form that they have learned are not effective. It only means that they are not effective in using them. A gun will certainly kill you, but first you have to hit the person with the bullet. So martial art techniques are definitely effective but first the person doing them must be able to hit the target with the right technique.

The martial arts are just that, art forms, and as such are beautiful to watch and tend to become a way of life with the true practioners. They are techniques that can be enjoyed and practiced for benefit by anyone, just as any great work of art can be enjoyed by all viewers.

The techniques found in this book do not just come from Karate, which is what many people think of when they hear the words martial arts, but they come from Judo, and Jiu-Jitsu, Kung Fu, Aikido, Kendo, Zen, Yoga, and even psychology and ballet. Techniques that can be applicable to all forms of sports have been utilized in this manual for the mutual benefit of the players and the fans. For no one wants to get hurt or see a player get hurt, and everyone wants maximum performance, a positive attitude and a stronger mind.

Let us examine the facts:

1. There is no better way in the world to learn how to fall without receiving an injury than to practice Judo falling techniques.

2. The most flexible people in the world are ballerinas and karate men. The stretches taken from these two arts will enable you to become as flexible as you wish.

3. There is only one art form in the world that teaches you how to get hit without getting injured: Jiu-Jitsu, and it does not require any magical mystical powers. It is simply breath, muscle and mind control all put together to form a new identity called KI. (Just like the various pieces of metal are all put together and form a new machine called a car.)

4. There is no better form or exercise to develop powers of concentration and mind control than techniques of meditation taken from Zen and Yoga.

5. Aikido is a 2,000 year old art form that enables one to overcome the largest of opponents with the minimal of effort by the use of balance points and leverage.

6. Breathing is both necessary to sustain life and vital in athletic performance, in relaxation and in concentration. If you don't believe me, hold your breath for a week, or try to sleep while breathing 70 times a minute. The best techniques of breath control in the world come from Yoga and its exercises.

7. The most powerful method of striking or hitting another person or thing ever developed comes from Karate techniques of weight shifting and striking. (Ever try to break a brick?)

8. Techniques of one sport can be applied to make other sports more effective.

So please do not find yourself being prejudiced against techniques found in this book before you even try them. They simply are the most effective means man has ever found to do the things described and if you will use them in your sport, you can improve your performance, develop a positive mental attitude and prevent most injuries. Keep an open mind, practice them and apply them in any way you wish. Adapt them to your style and use them at your discretion, but employ them and use them and you and your sport will greatly benefit.

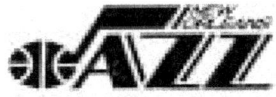

P. O. BOX 5303 • NEW ORLEANS, LOUISIANA 70150 • (504) 581-4055

September 30, 1977

Mr. Ted Gambordella
P. O. Box 1288
Alexandria, Louisiana 71301

Dear Ted:

On behalf of the New Orleans Jazz, I want to thank you for being of great
assistance in our pre-season training program. The Jazz put a great deal
of emphasis on pre-season training and conditioning and have always been
on the lookout for new techniques and new ideas in this area. We were
most fortunate to learn of you and persuade you to assist us.

The period of time you spent with our team in pre-season has been invaluable.
Your relaxation techniques and stretching muscle exercises are still being
done each day by our players. This is the first pre-season period in our
short history we have not had the usual muscle pulls and sprains of the
past. We can only attribute that to your program.

After you left, I had informal conversations with each of our players concerning
the time spent with you. Each and everyone felt that what you had taught
them concerning their bodies and how their bodies react to stress was, not only
meaningful, but something they plan to use from here on in. Even though some
of our players put more emphasis on different areas of your teachings, each
one to a number felt they got something out of each of your sessions. They,
the players, are the toughest critics and most difficult to fool when it comes
to their bodies. You have passed the test.

We look forward to having you with us next year to work with our players, not
only on the techniques that you demonstrated this year, but anything new which
you believe will be of help to our team. Thank you once again for your
patience, your help and your ideas.

In friendship,

NEW ORLEANS JAZZ

Lewis Schaffel
General Manager

LS/mc

Oklahoma State University

DEPARTMENT OF ATHLETICS

STILLWATER, OKLAHOMA 74074
GALLAGHER HALL
(405) 624-3645

November 10, 1977

TO WHOM IT MAY CONCERN:

I recently spent the afternoon with Mr. Ted Gambordella discussing his ideas concerning injury prevention, flexibility and relaxation techniques. I definitely feel his ideas would be of great benefit in our wrestling program and plan further sessions with Ted.

I was particularly interested in balance techniques and mind control techniques and how they can be related to wrestling. I also felt his techniques of breath control and breathing will be very useful for the team in the area of quick recovery and better performance.

I definitely recommend Ted Gambordella and his program of injury prevention to all coaches and wrestlers.

Sincerely,

Tommy Chesbro

Tommy Chesbro
Head Wrestling Coach

TC:jl

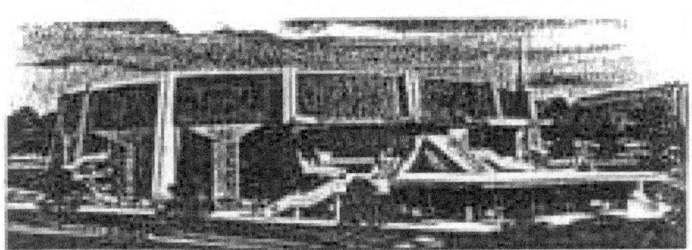

Oral Roberts University Department of Intercollegiate Athletics

7777 South Lewis
Tulsa, Oklahoma 74105
Phone (918) 492-2510

November 10, 1977

To Whom It May Concern,

Our basketball team had the privilege recently of having Mr. Ted Gambordella spend a few days with us. His presentation was excellent and his many ideas relating to injuries, flexibility, concentration, and relaxation are very applicable for use in athletics.

I was impressed with his knowledge and high quality presentation. I would highly recommend his presentation to any team, trainer or sports organization.

Sincerely,

Lake Kelly
Lake Kelly
Head Basketball Coach
Oral Roberts University

LK/dh

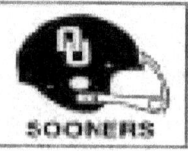

SOONERS

The University of Oklahoma
180 West Brooks   Room 221   Norman, Oklahoma 73019

February 28, 1979

To Whom It May Concern:

After working with Ted Gambordella and his program of injury prevention I feel that this program has many beneficial areas that can be of use in helping to prevent football injuries.

I was impressed with the balance point techniques and the KI-taing punches and elbows in the ribs and stomach. The following techniques also proved beneficial and we plan to use applicable techniques in our program.

I recommend Ted and his program to any coach or trainer to help prevent injuries.

Sincerely,

Barry Switzer
Head Football Coach

BS/kd

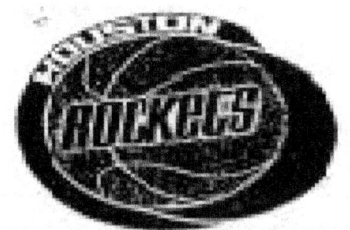

national basketball association

To whom it may concern:

Mr. Ted Gambordella recently spent some time with our basketball team and taught his course of injury prevention.

I felt the course was of definite benefit to our team and could be a factor in helping our team to stay healthy.

The team members felt the course was very worthwhile and intend to employ many of the techniques taught in the class as part of their regular program.

I feel Mr. Gambordella's program can be of benefit to any professional or amateur coach and team and I highly recommend him and his program.

Sincerely,

Tom Nissalke
Head Coach

TN/se

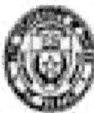

THE UNIVERSITY OF TEXAS AT AUSTIN
MEN'S INTERCOLLEGIATE ATHLETICS
AUSTIN, TEXAS 78712

Office of The
Head Football Coach

November 3, 1977

TO WHOM IT MAY CONCERN:

Mr. Ted Gambordella has recently spent time with our
football squad. His ideas concerning injury prevention,
we feel will be very helpful to our football team. He
also has some outstanding programs for flexibility,
relaxation and improving leverage and balance points.
I definitely feel that adopting Mr. Gambordella's ideas
will help our program and we plan to have him continue
working with us.

Yours truly,

Fred Akers

af

LOUISIANA STATE UNIVERSITY

AND AGRICULTURAL AND MECHANICAL COLLEGE
BATON ROUGE   *   LOUISIANA   *   70803

Basketball Office

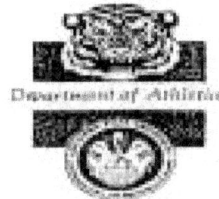

Department of Athletics

September 9, 1977

TO WHOM IT MAY CONCERN:

During the past month I have had the opportunity to observe
Mr. Ted Gambordella, while he has worked with our basketball
players in an advanced fitness and strength class which they
are currently enrolled in at L.S.U. He has certainly captured
their attention and belief in his fantastic ability of the
mastery of the mind.

In my opinion, Ted Gambordella has the possibilities of open-
ing a new dimension in college athletics with many of his
techniques and I think can prove to be a fantastic asset to
any program.

Ted is most knowledgeable and comes across with an assurance
of himself in what he is teaching and has been most impressive
to me during the past month. It has been a most worthwhile and
educational experience for our L.S.U. basketball players to have
worked under Mr. Gambordella and I am confident his theories
will pay great dividends to us once the season starts.

If you would like any further information about Mr. Gambordella
and his program, please feel free to contact me at any time,
as I would be happy to recommend Ted Gambordella and his program
to anyone.

Sincerely,

Dale D. Brown
Head Basketball Coach

DDB:pk

ATHLETIC DEPARTMENT

October 24, 1977

To Whom It May Concern:

Mr. Ted Gambordella worked with the Rice University Football Team for one week. He taught us techniques in preventing athletic injuries that has definitely helped our football team.

His classes included very valuable techniques for the team on stretching, balance points, relaxation, how to get hit without being injured, and falling.

Our players expressed many positive reactions that the classes definitely helped them for the future of their football career. I believe the classes were instrumental in helping us develop techniques that can be used in our off season program to develop strength, quickness, flexibility, and endurance.

Without reservations, I recommend Ted Gambordella's injury prevention program for other teams.

Sincerely,

HOMER C. RICE
Director of Athletics and
Head Football Coach

HCR/jb

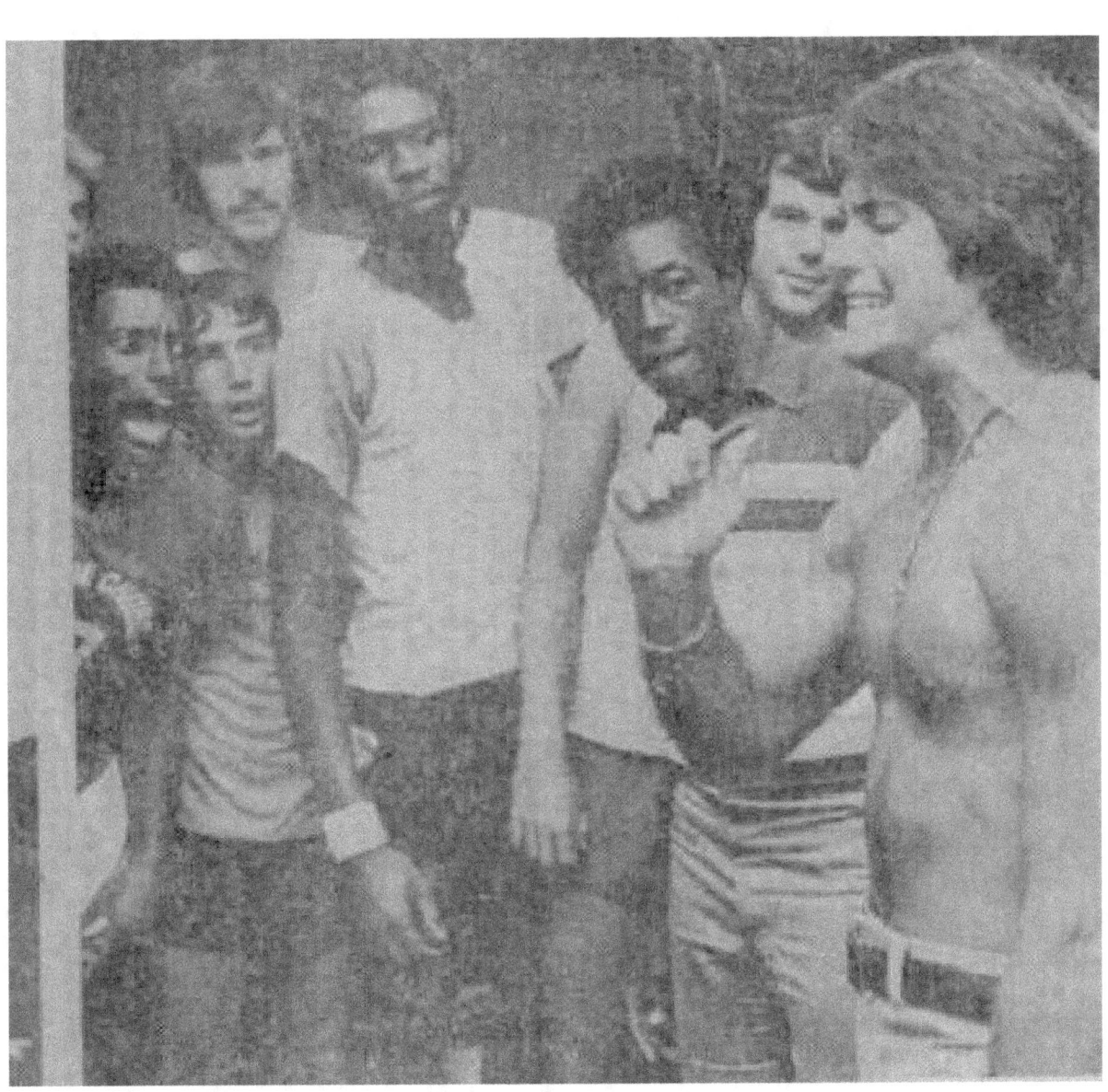

TABLE OF CONTENTS

Chapter 1

FLEXIBILITY

The importance of flexibility as a factor in preventing athletic injuries, and improving performance cannot be overemphasized. It is a fact that the flexibility of the athlete plays a vital factor in the reduction of leg injuries, the increase of the player's own body control and the improvement of performance due to the increase of mobility and coordination. Such injuries as a pulled hamstring, a pulled groin, or a sprained ankle are much less likely to occur when the athlete has adequate flexibility. In fact, many professional teams now employ a full time flexibility coach to help assure full performance and to reduce flexibility related injuries.

There is a vast difference between a muscle being "stretched" and a "limber" muscle. Once a muscle has been truly "stretched" it will tend to remain so over a great period of time. It is like folding a piece of paper, once the fold has been made the paper will always have a crease in it. So once a muscle has been stretched it will always have the tendency to remain so. A muscle that has only been limbered up is one that will quickly snap back to its shorten state, and thereby increase the chances of a flexibility related injury.

The proper method for performing a stretching program is to take your time and allow the muscles to gradually lengthen as you bend, not bounce or jerk in your movements. It is virtually impossible to loosen up and truly stretch a muscle in 10 seconds (a condition you often see athletes trying to perform as the coach calls them off the bench into the game).

If the athlete goes into the game cold, or not fully limber or stretched, then he is going to have to use a few minutes of the actual game time to get loose enough for his top performance. This could mean giving up a first down or missing a block, a tackle, blowing a shot, etc. So the athlete should strive to stay stretched on the side lines by doing a few simple stretches while he is sitting on the bench, standing on the sidelines or even waiting between plays.

To get the fullest stretch, the muscle must be warm. Therefore, if the athlete is stretching in the winter, he should wear long pants or a sweat suit while stretching. If it is warm in the summer, shorts are appropriate. Care should be taken to make sure that the muscles do not become cold and stiff during the game or practice session. So the athlete should always be trying to stay loose.

In all of these stretches where you are trying to make a maximum effort or bend, try to hold the point of full extension between 5 and 15 seconds.

Flexibility

One of the most important Martial Arts Fitness Secrets is FLEXIBILITY. If you are not flexible, you look and feel 10 years older than you should. Flexibility allows you to participate in activities and do things like a 20 year old.

Back pain is often caused by lack of flexibility. This lack of flexibility often causes the back to tighten up when exercising, thus causing muscle pulls and stiffness that easily could be avoided with a few simple stretches.

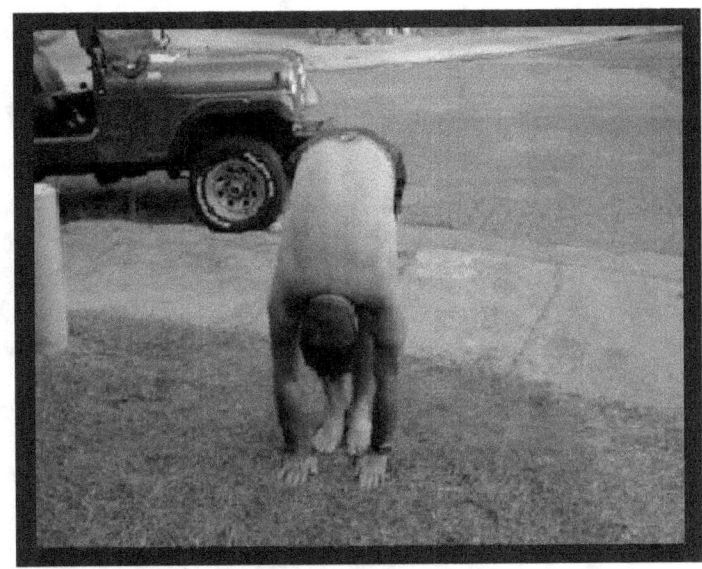

How often should you stretch. Everyday until you feel loose, and every time before you begin a strenuous exercise. Even if you only do your stretches for 3 to 5 minutes this is better than pulling a muscle or tearing a muscle because you didn't take the time to loosen up.

Here are some simple flexibility exercises you can do every day to keep the body fluid.

Trunk Rotation

Place your hands on your
hips and rotate the body in
large circles to the right and
left.
Do about 10 turns clockwise,
and then 10 turn counter
clockwise.

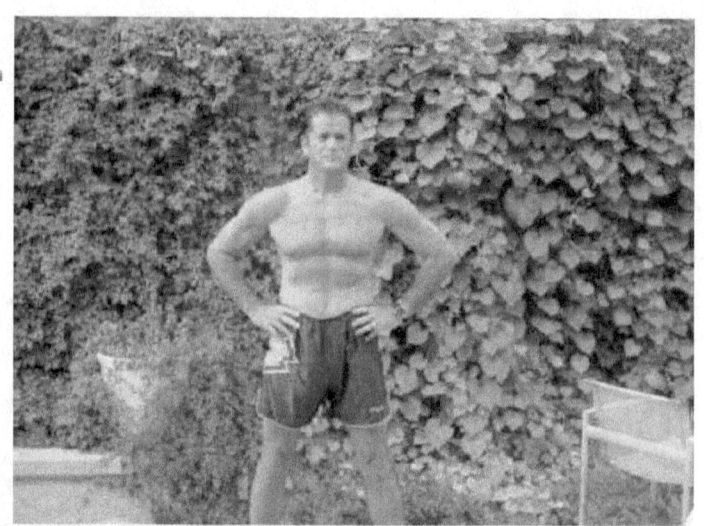

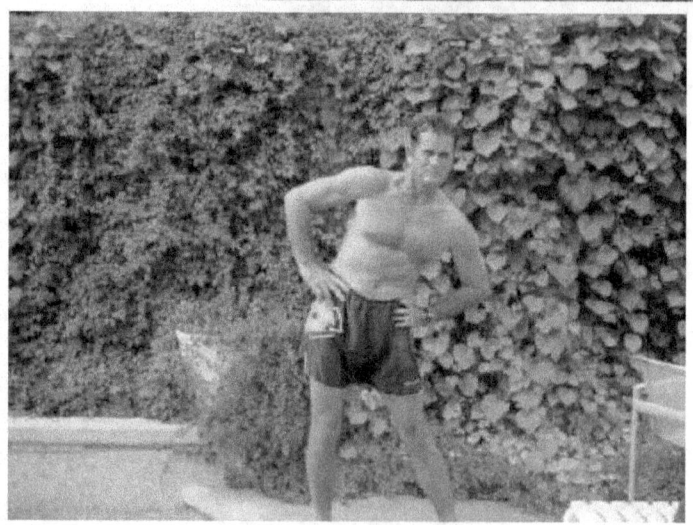

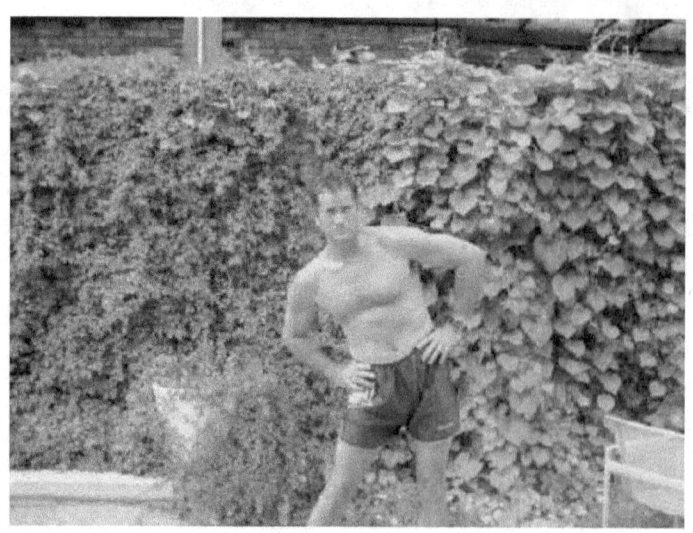

BODY TWISTS

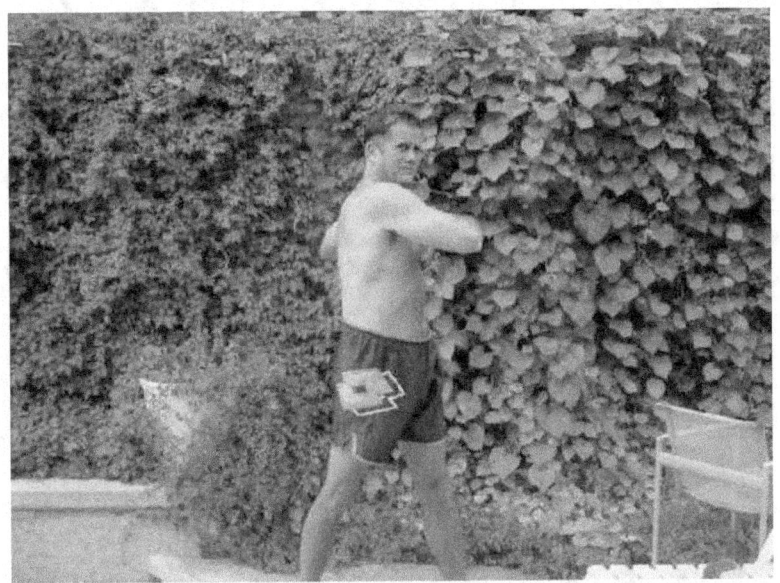

Pull the elbows up to shoulder height
and twist hard to the left and right.

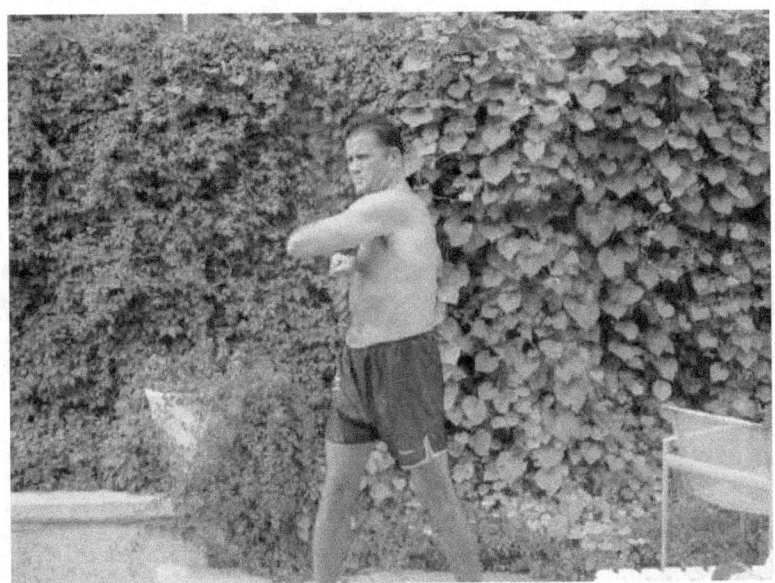

Do 10 to 12 twists to each side

ARM CIRCLES

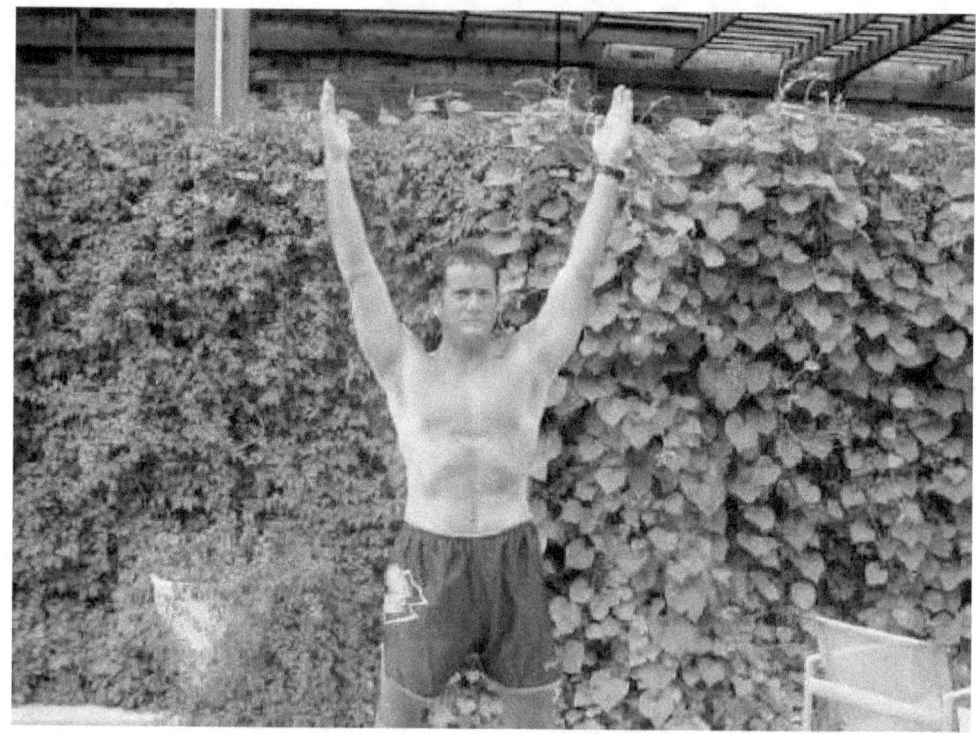

Swing the arms in large circles around the body. Forward and backwards

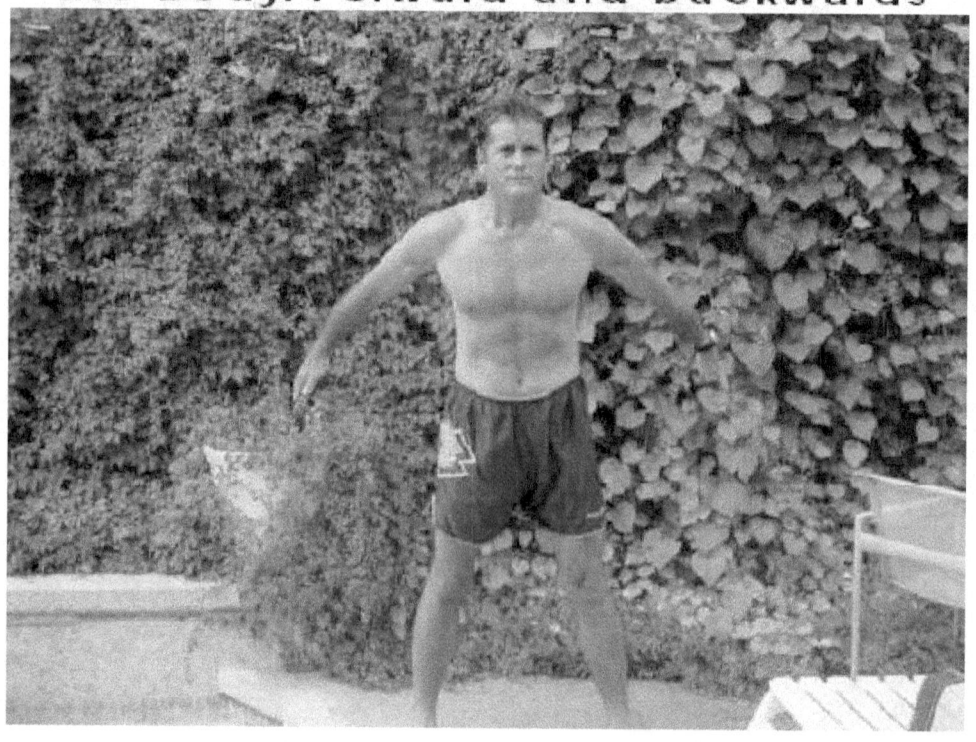

Do about 10 to 12 swings each direction

NECK CIRCLES
&
SHOULDER SHRUGS

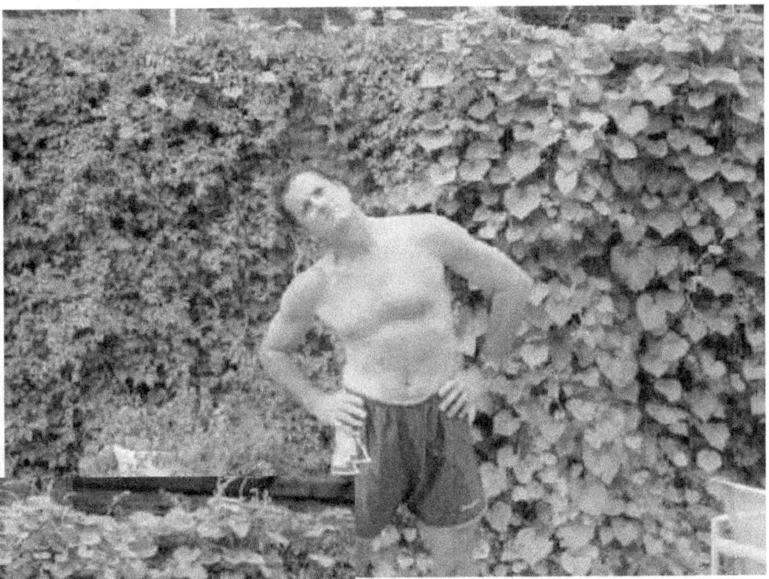

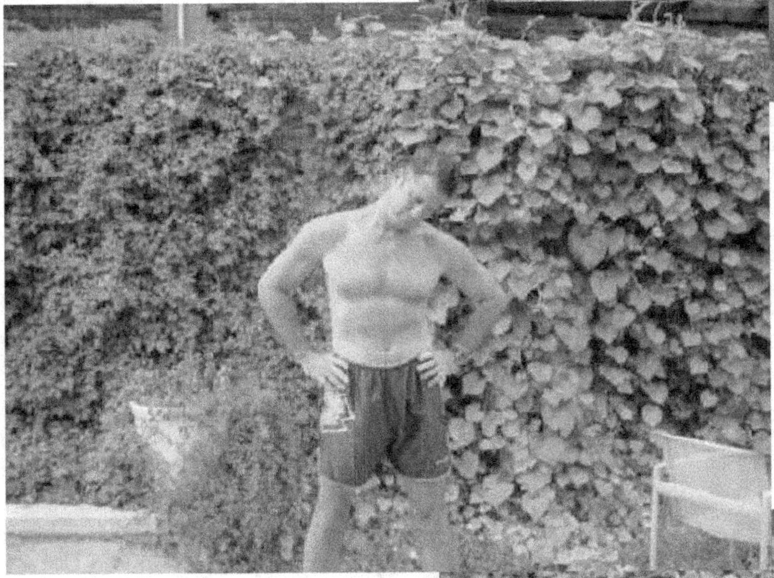

Rotate the neck
in small circles
clockwise and
counter clockwise
Do about 10 - 12

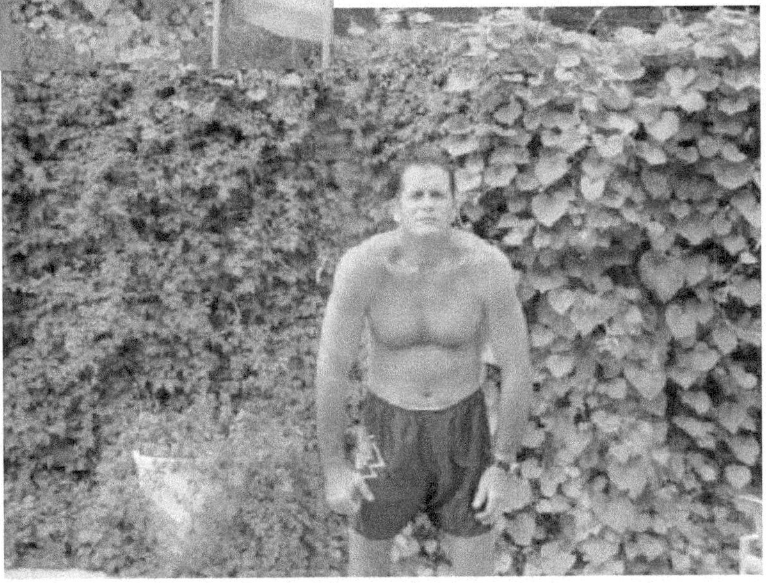

Shrug the shoulders
in circles forward
and backwards
10 - 12 times

Horse Stretch

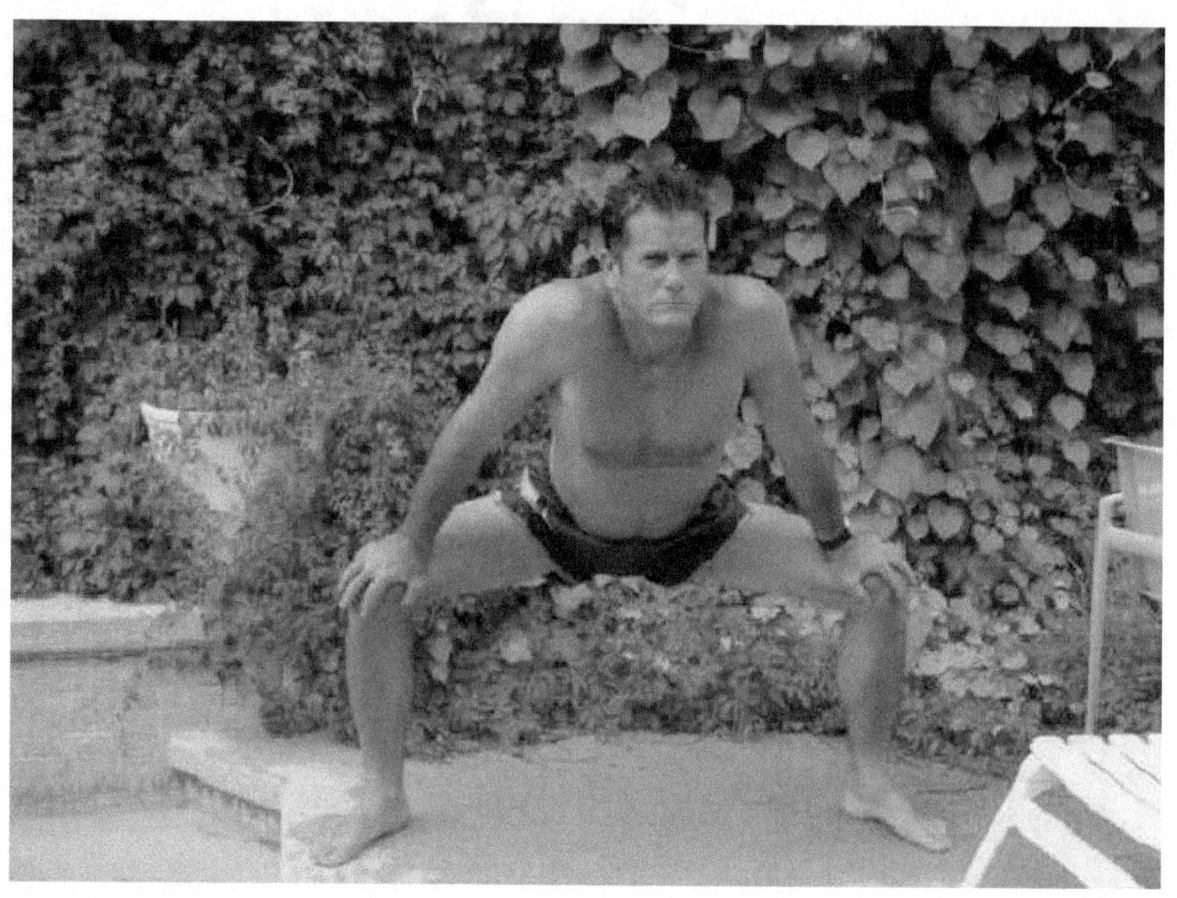

Squat very low and push the hips down
into the squat. Move from side to side
and then drop to the ground on each side.

Do 10 - 12 times each side

W STRETCHES

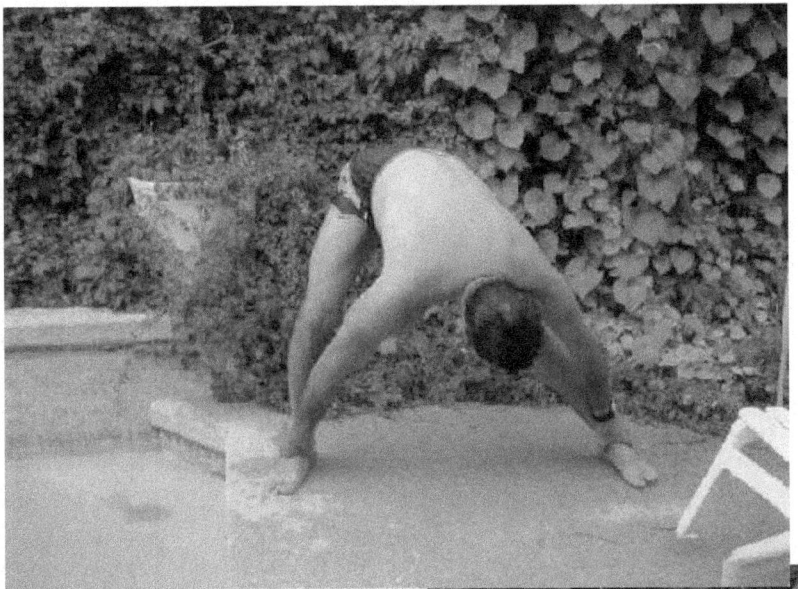

Lean over and grab the ankles. Drop to one side and try to straighten the leg. Then the other side.
Now pull the head down to the knee, then over to the other knee.
Finally drop down in the middle and try to touch the head to the ground.

You can also drop the elbows to the ground

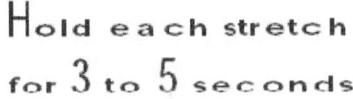

Hold each stretch for 3 to 5 seconds

BUTTERFLY

Hold the ankles and try to get the knees down to the ground. You may bounce, and push down with the elbows.

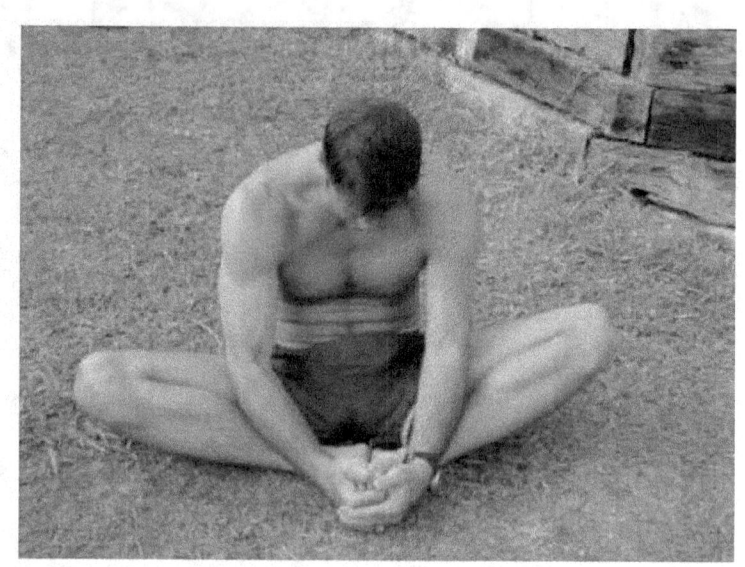

STRAIGHT LEGGED STRETCH

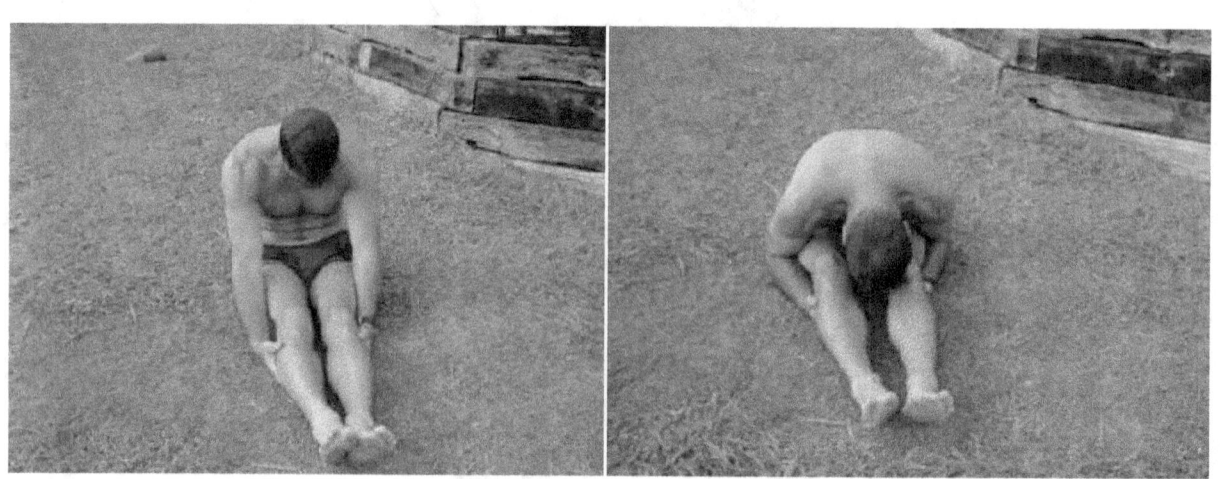

Keep the legs straight and hold the knees.
Try to pull the head down till it touches the knees.
Hold for 3 to 5 seconds. Do this 10 times.

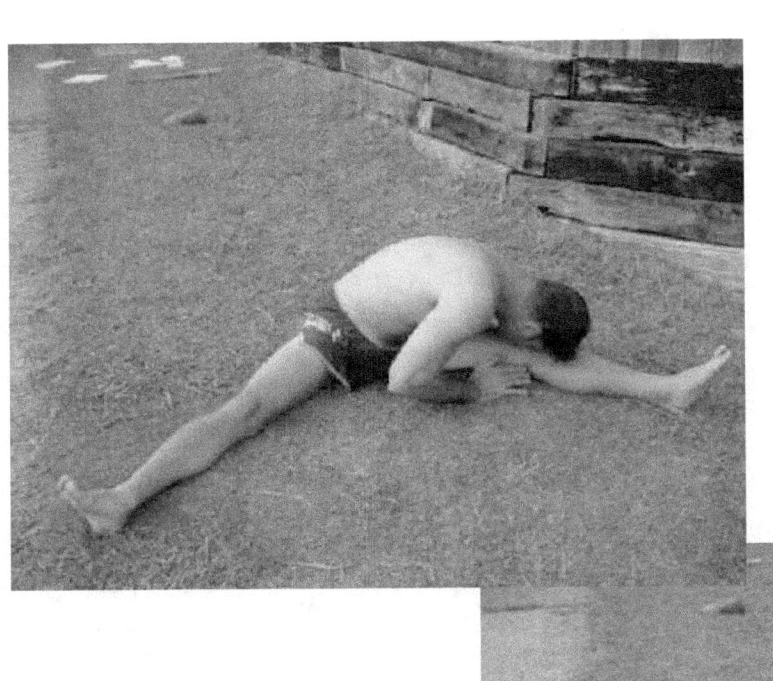

V STRETCH

Sit on the ground and spread the legs as wide as you can. Now lean to the right and touch the head to the knee, then the left.
Finish touching the head to the ground in the middle.

If you are having trouble touching your head to the ground it is not your legs or back that is the problem. It is your Hips. The next exercise will help loosen your hips.

HIP STRETCH

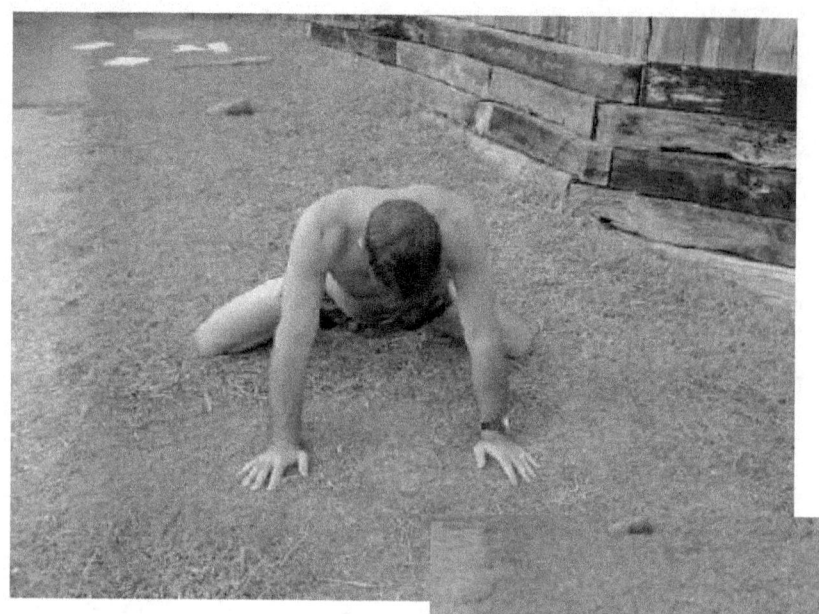

Open your legs as wide as possible and try to force the knees and hips to the ground.

You can start with your hand stiff then as you loosen up drop to your elbows and finally touch the head and hips to the ground

You can bounce on this stretch. Hold the final position for 5 to 10 seconds.

AMERICAN SPLITS

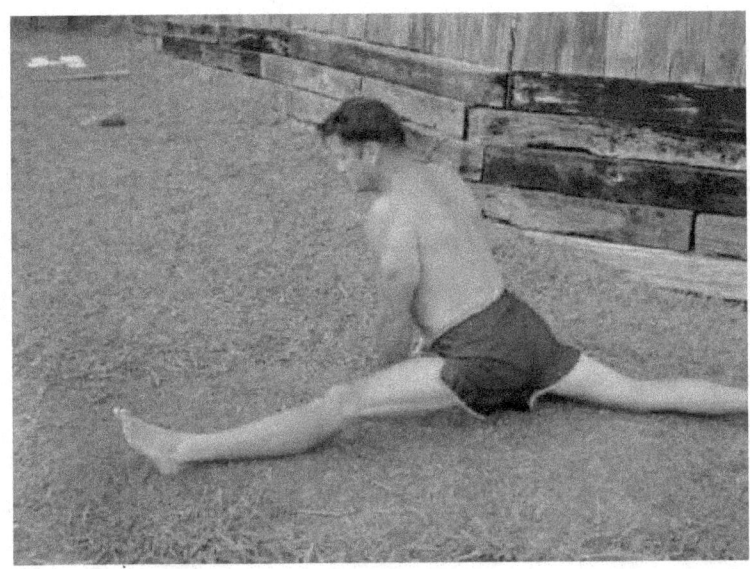

To really stretch the hips you should push hard to do the American Splits. Spread the legs as wide as possible directly in front of the body. Try to touch the hips to the ground.

You can use your hands to help support your body weight, and you may lean forward to drop the hips ddown.

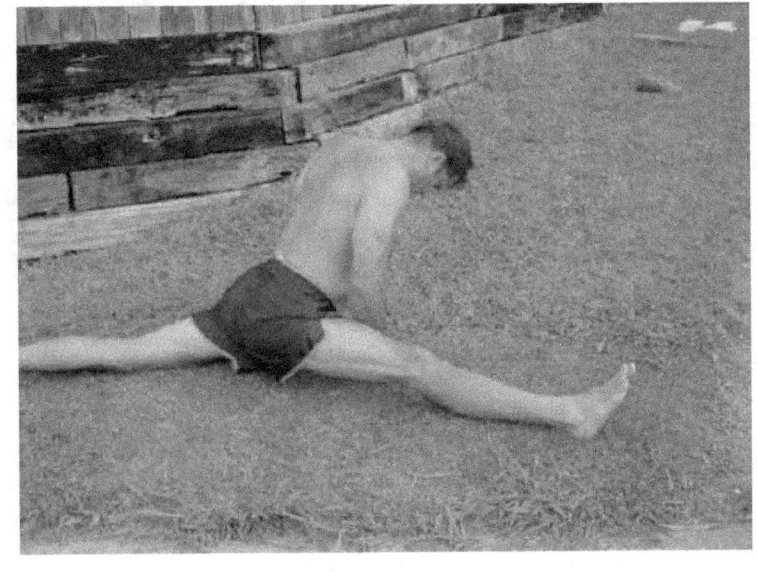

BACK STRETCH

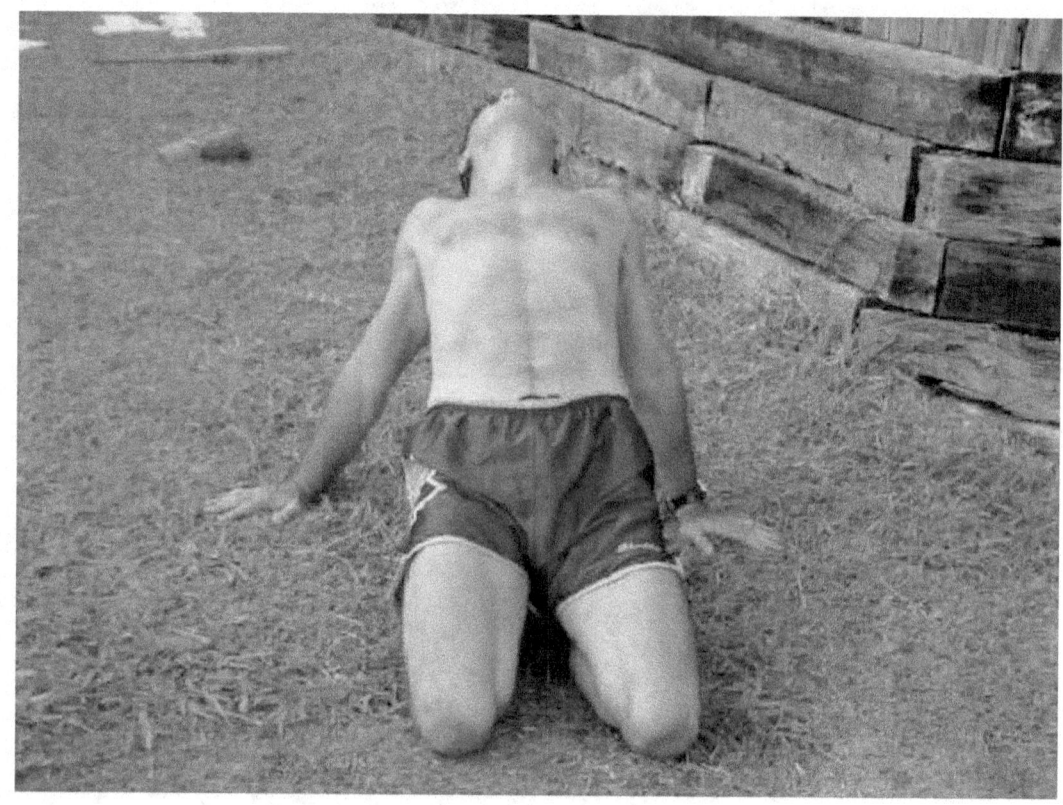

Sit on the legs and bend backwards as
Far as you can comfortably go. Use your hands for
support. You do not have to go all the way back.

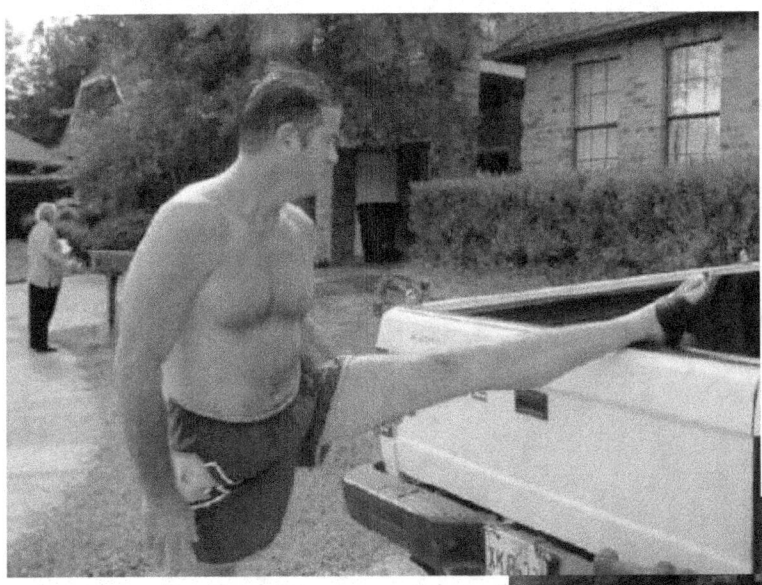

BAR STRETCHING

Bar Stretching is great, but most people don't have a bar in their home or gym. So you can use a truck, or car back, or even a table.

Put your leg on the truck back, and lean over to touch the head to the knees. Do both side. Hold each stretch 5 seconds.

You can also lean To the right and left to put more pressure on the stretching leg.

BAR STRETCHING 2

Put the leg on a low table and drop the weight down to stretch the hamstrings. Keep the leg straight.

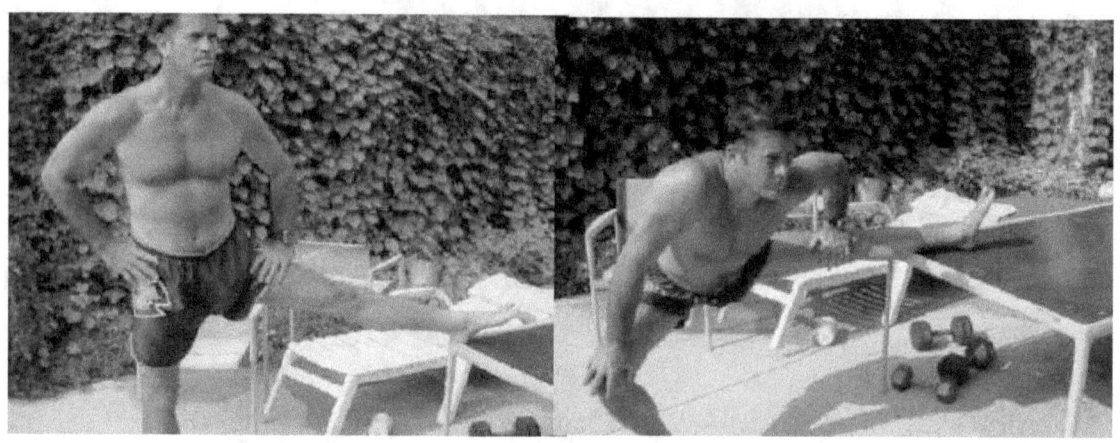

Lean over and touch the head to the knee. Do both legs

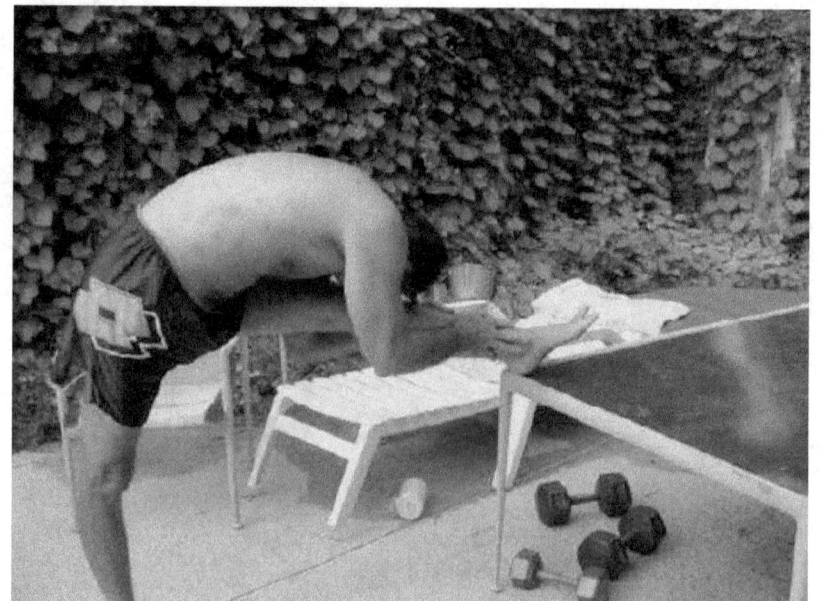

HIP AND KNEE STRETCH

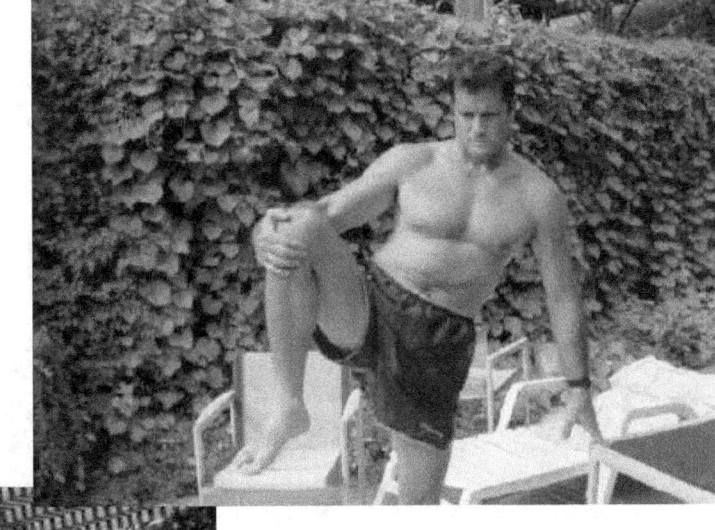

Keep the back straight and lift the knee as high as you can to the side. Pull up on the knee and stretch the back of th legs.

Now drop the knee down and pull back on the leg. To stretch the front of th legs

Pull back as far as you can and you may lean over into the table.

STRETCHING WITH A PARTNER

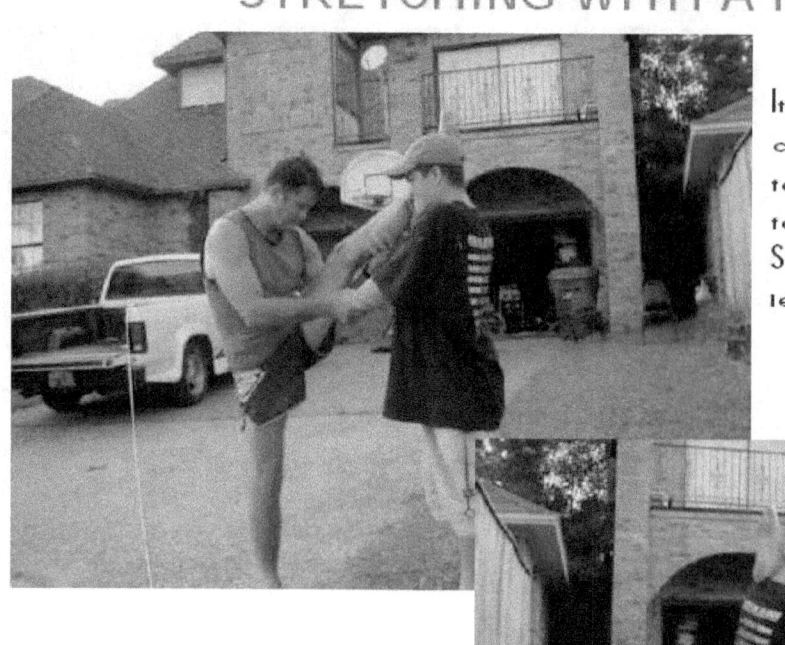

If you have a partner. You can hold on to their hand for balance and place your foot on their shoulder. Stretch forward. Do both legs.

You can also lean down and drop your weight to put more stretch on your leg

PARTNER STRETCH 2

Hold on the wall for support and have your partner stretch your leg straight up.

Side stretch. Lean to the side and have the partner stretch the leg up like your doing a side kick

Try to straighten your body up as much as possible into the stretch.

PARTNER BACK STRETCH

Have the partner hold your arms by the elbows and lean backwards. He will gently pick you up and stretch your back. Go

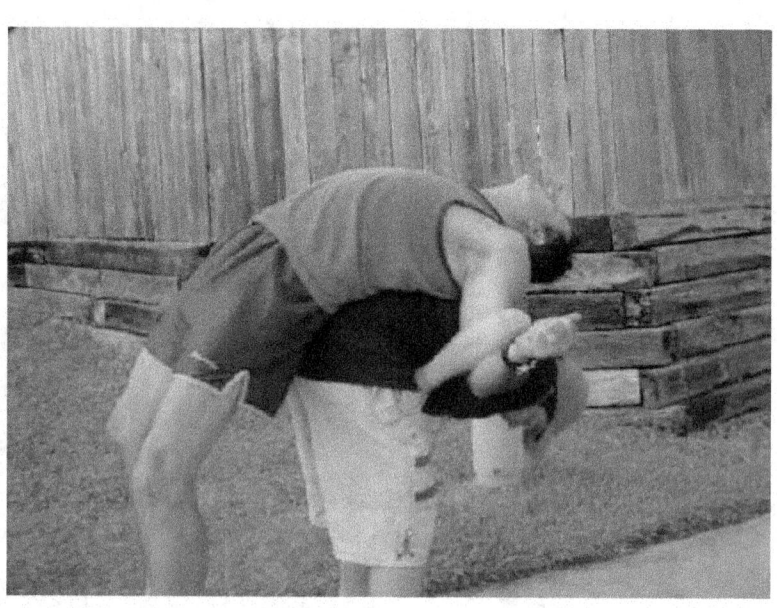

PARTNER SHOULDER STRETCH

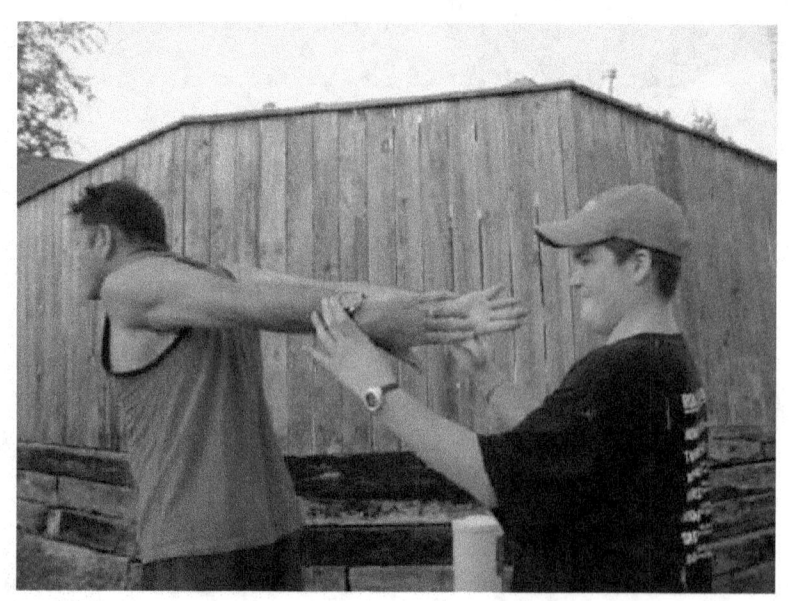

Have your partner pull your arms straight back across your body to stretch the shoulders. Go slow and easy.

Martial Arts Secrets of Fitness
Weight Training

Weight Training is an important part of Martial Arts Fitness Training and is something that should be done consistently throughout your entire life. You are never too old to start lifting weights, but you can be too young. I do not suggest that you let a child whom has not reached puberty to lift weights. Wait until the child is at least 13 and then only lift what they can comfortably handle. Do not force them to do heavy reps. Let them build up their muscles. It is important not to turn the child off to weight training so that they will want to continue to lift their entire lives.

I lift weights every other day for 6 days, then take off Sunday. On the days I do not lift weights I walk, do karate, wrestle, golf, or some other form of hard aerobic exercise. When I walk, or golf I always carry a weight in my hands. This doubles the exercise effectiveness by allowing an arm and upper body workout, while working out the legs, abs and heart with the walking or golf.

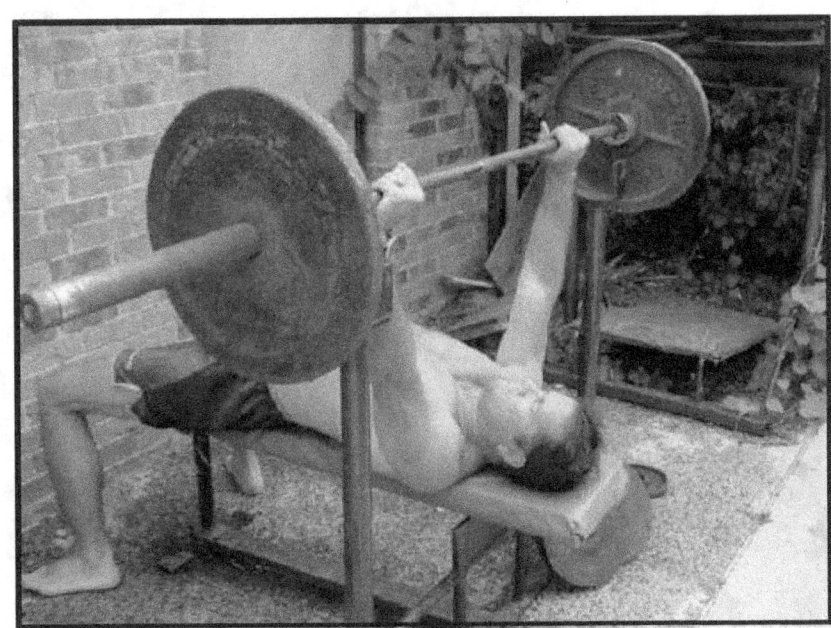

I do not lift Heavy weights. I am 54 years old and do not need to try to bench 300 pounds to prove I am strong or build my chest. I already have a great chest and keep it toned and pumped by lifting smaller weights, but lifting them hundreds of times.

I work out on the bench with 135 pounds, or 2 big plates and do reps of 50 to 100. 50 to 100 times for each set.

BENCH PRESS

The Bench Press is one of my favorite exercises. It works the entire chest, shoulders, back, and abs. I do a lot of bench presses.

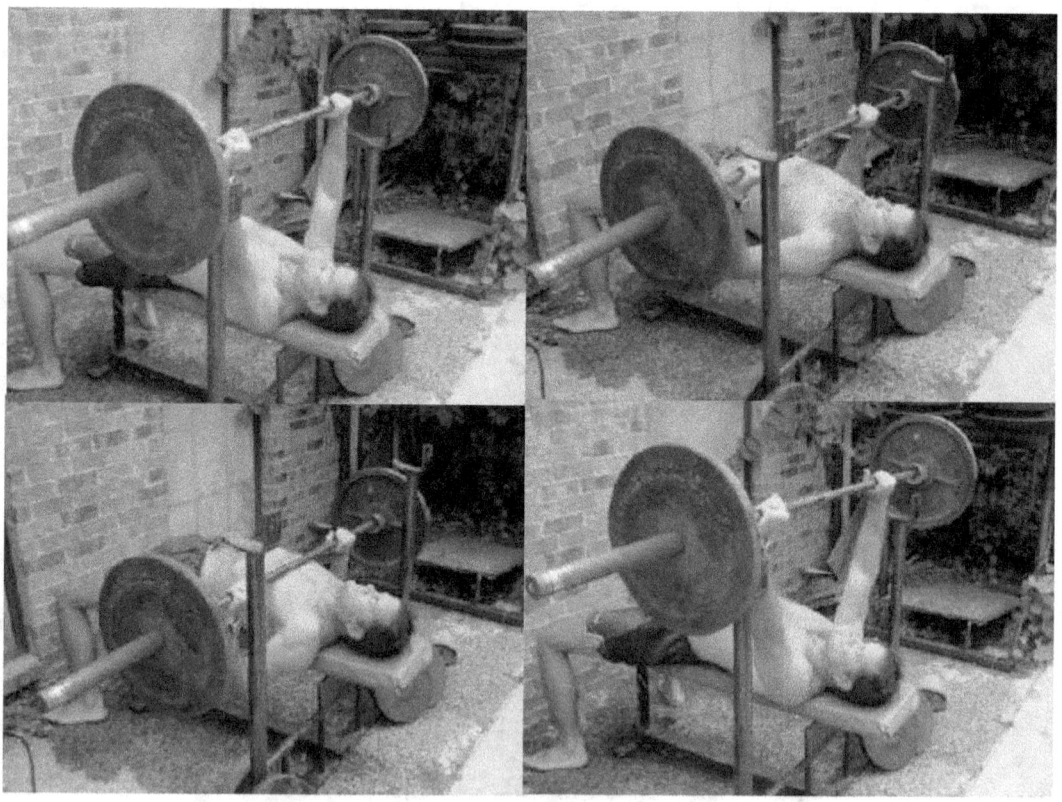

To do the regular bench press grasp the bar with the hands evenly spaced. Lower the bar slowly to the chest and hold it about 1 second then push it back up to the top. I warm up with 2 sets of about 10 "full" lifting reps.

This is the last set of "full" lifts I do. After my warm ups I go to my "modified" or "half up" bench press and do 6 to 10 sets of 50 to 100.

MODIFIED BENCH PRESS
Narrow Hands

During these sets I keep my hands a little narrow about the width of my chest and I DO NOT LIFT the bar all the way back up. I Pump the Chest by only lifting the bar Half Way Up and then back down.

I bring the bar down to the chest, but only about ½ way back up. This allows me to pump the chest up by the large amounts of reps I do.

I do 5 to 10 sets of 50 to 100 reps. That is not a mistype. I do 50 to 100 reps for 5 to 10 sets.

MODIFIED BENCH PRESS
Wide Hands

Here I do the same half up reps but now my hands are very wide and I drop the weight more towards my neck.

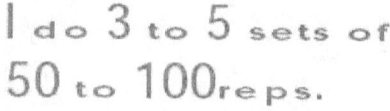

I do 3 to 5 sets of 50 to 100 reps.

MODIFIED BENCH PRESS
REVERSE Hands

Here I reverse the
position of my
hands and do half
ups. The reverse
hands works my
triceps more and
the lower chest.

I do 2 to 4 sets of
20 to 40 reps.

INCLINE PRESS

The Incline Press is a better exercise for building a large beautiful chest than the bench. It works the upper pecs and shoulders and gives the chest a full and hard look that is not achieved by doing flat bench. I do a lot of inclines and for many years only did inclines with very little flat bench.

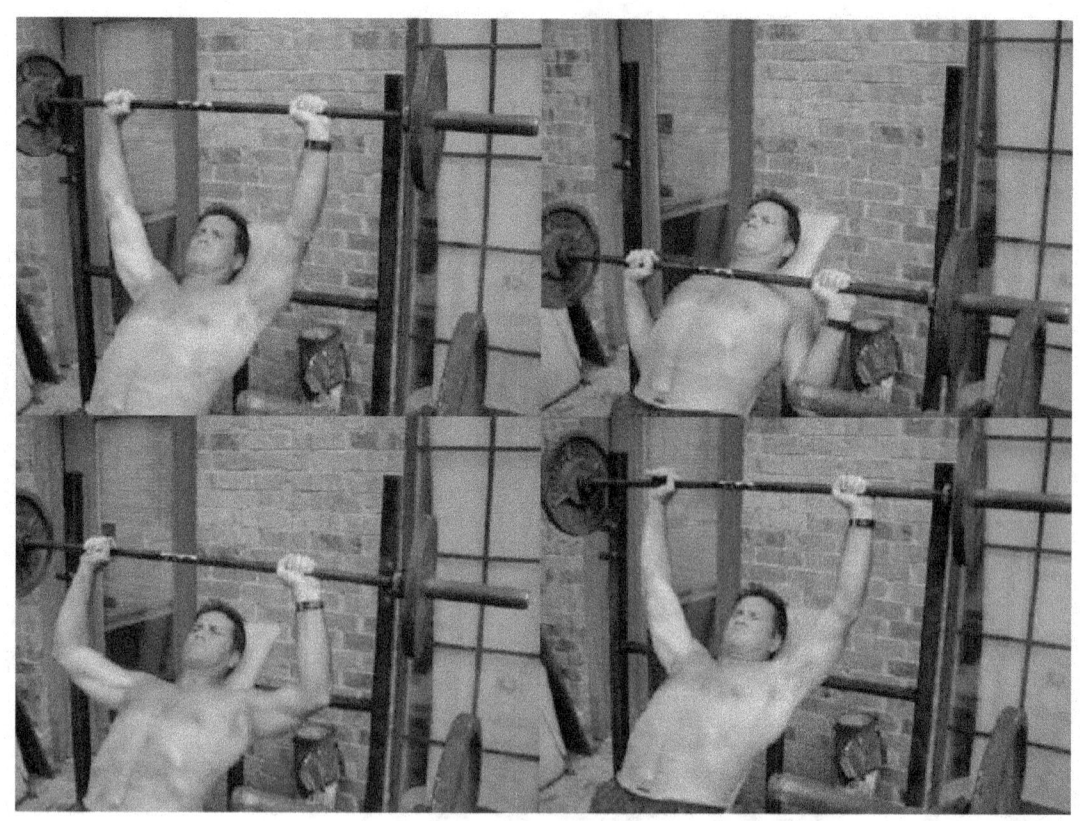

Warm up doing ful extension reps. 2 sets of 10 to 15 reps.

INCLINE PRESS
NARROW GRIP

Here I grip the bar with my hand about as wide as my chest and I use a "half up" motion. I do not go all the up. I only go about 5 to 12 inches.

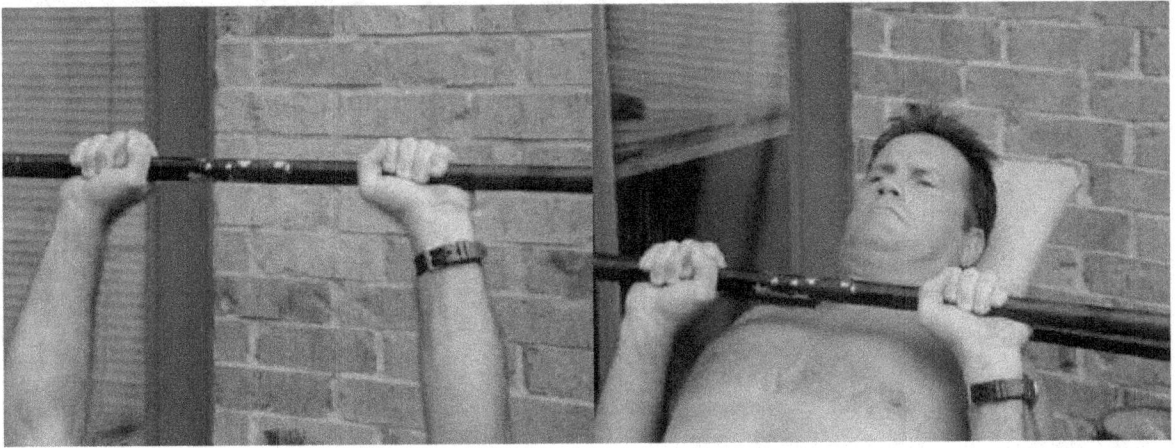

I do 5 to 8 sets of 35 to 75. It is important to watch your breathing because you can easily run out of breath doing inclines. Be sure to breath every few reps. And it is also important to have a "spotter" to help lift the bar off your chest if you are forcing the last few reps. Unlike the flat bench. You really can't cheat and put the bar up on the incline. When your chest is exhausted you will need help to put the bar up.

INCLINE PRESS
Wide GRIP

Here once again I do not go all the way up, I use half ups and go about 6 to 12 inches. I do 4 sets of 35 to 50.

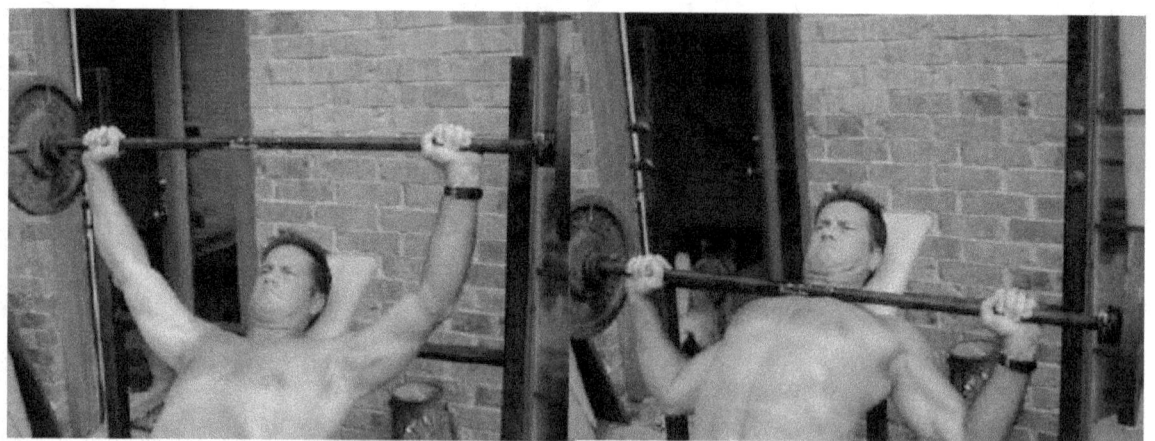

SQUATS

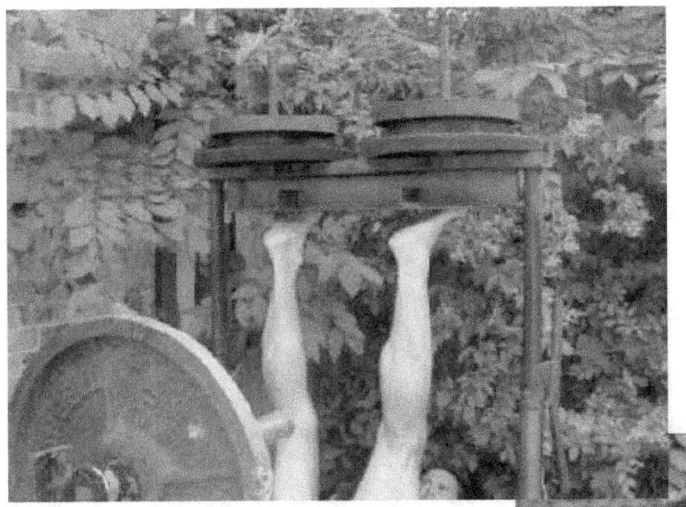

Let me say that I do not advocate doing squats with the bar on your back. This has always hurt my back and will wind up hurting yours. You can get the same results doing the squats from your back, or on a "hack" squat machine, where you lie on your back and the rack is about 45% up.

You can do the full squat and when you are thru, do some toe raises to work the caffs.

I do 6 sets of 20 to 40 reps.

DUMBELLS

Regular Curls

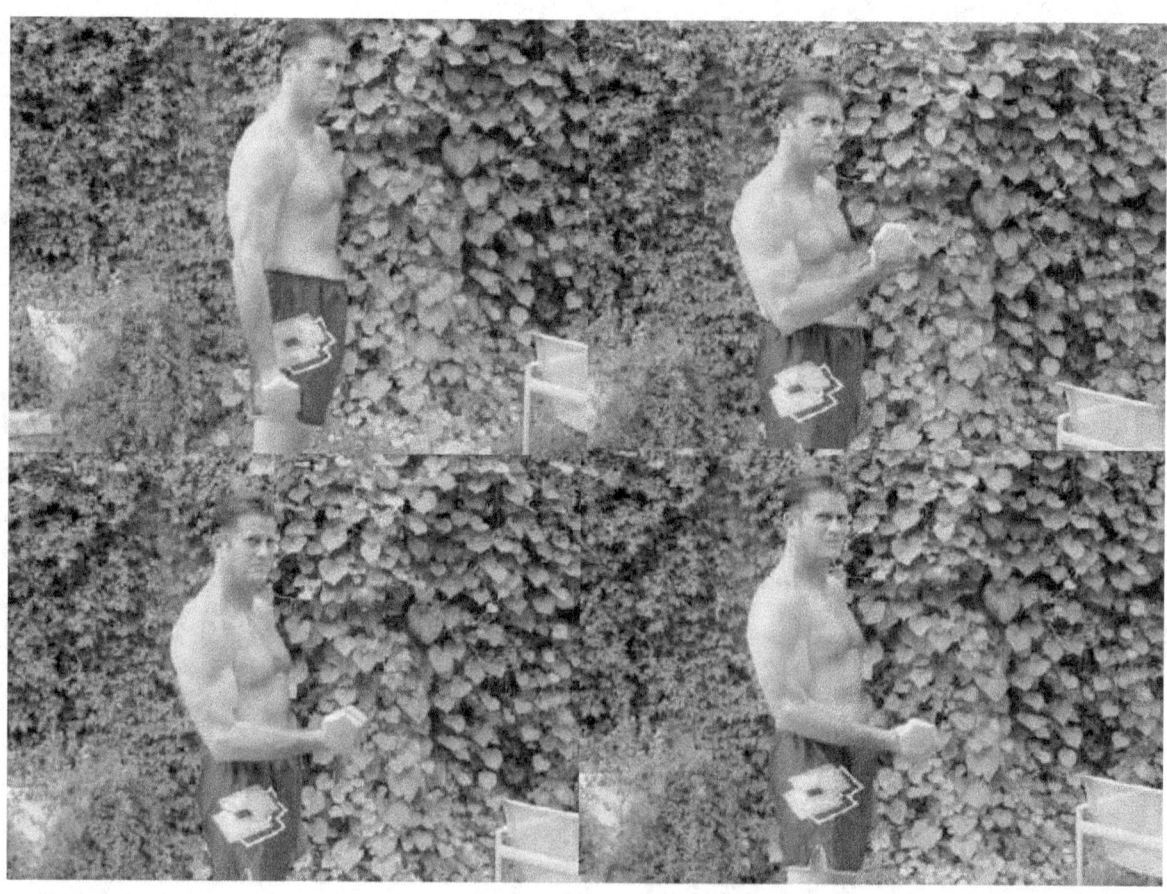

Stand with the feet about shoulder width apart and curl the weight straight up. I alternate arms, and one arm at a time so I can concentrate on the exercise.
Do 6 sets of 12 to 24 reps.

DUMBELLS

Cross overs

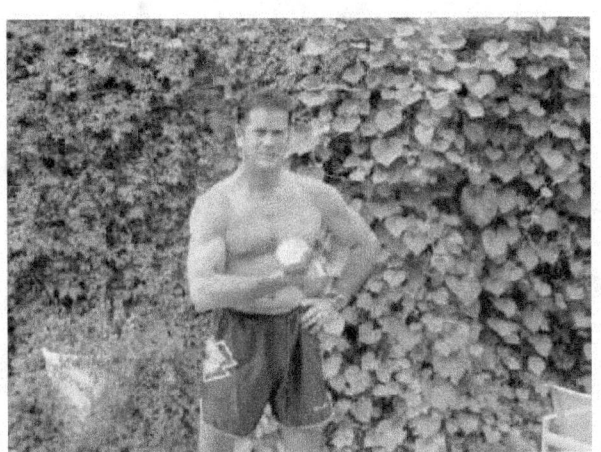 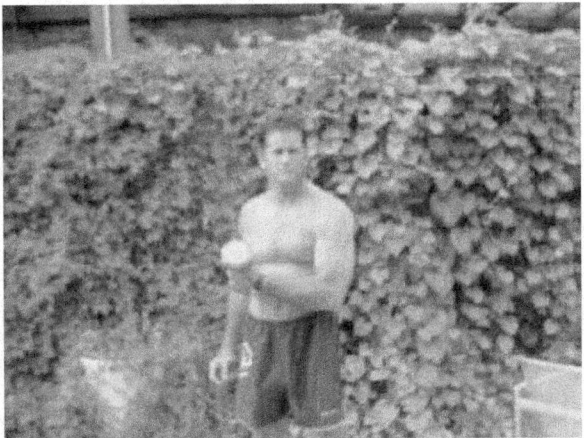

Stand with the feet about shoulder width apart and curl the weight up and across the body. You can alternate arms, or use weights in both hands. Turn the weight over as you curl up.

Do 4 sets of 12 to 16 reps.

DUMBELLS

Straight curls heavy weight

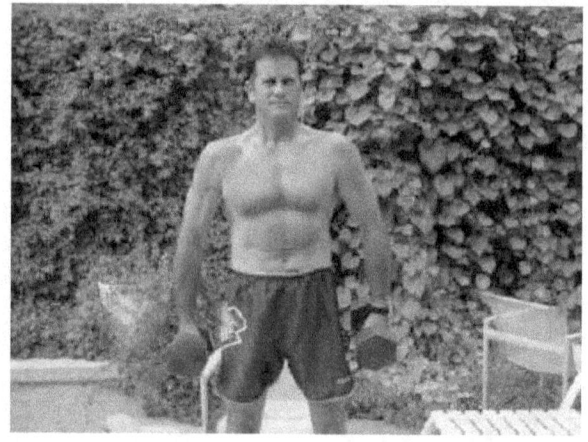 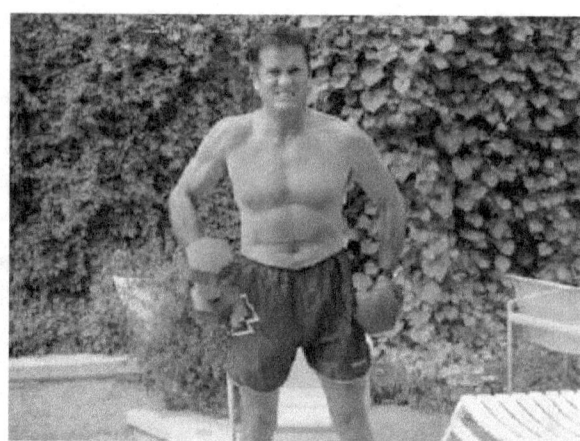

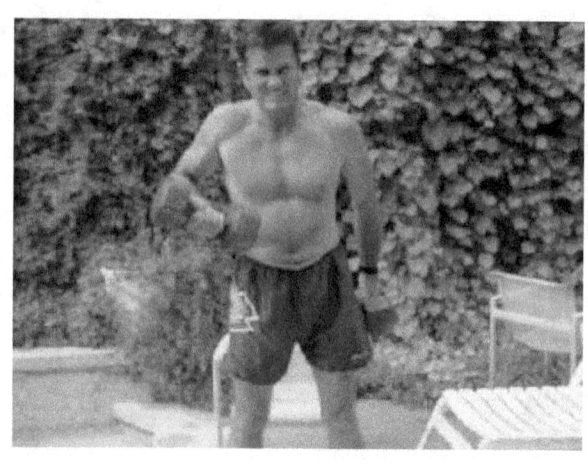 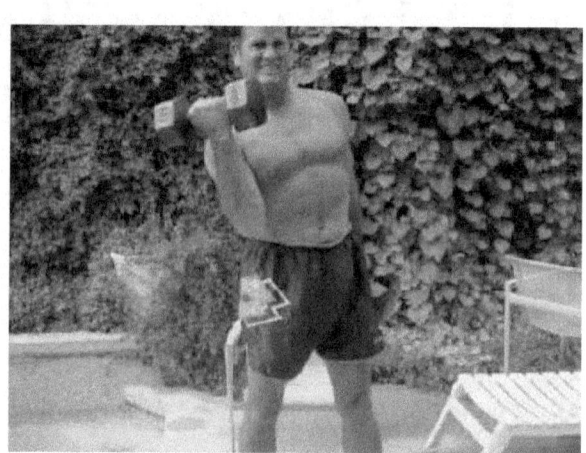

This curl is done raising the arm straight up and curling the weight. I use heavy weights and really push the body to build the muscle. So I do less reps.

Do 4 sets of 4 to 6 reps.

DUMBELLS

Triceps extensions

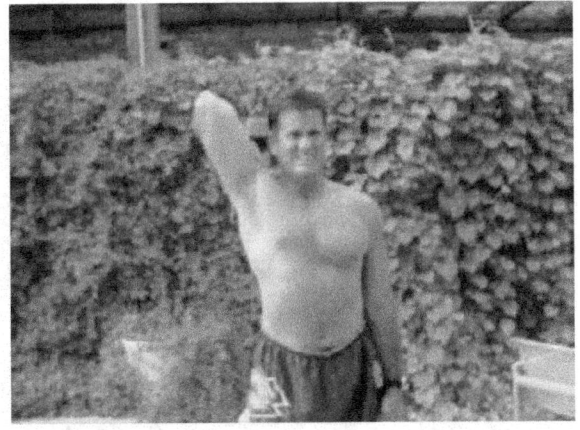
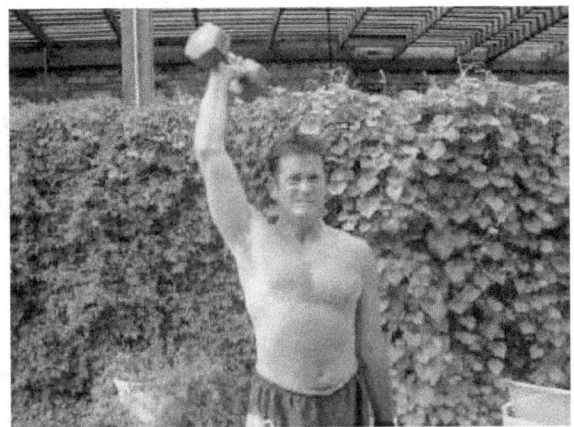
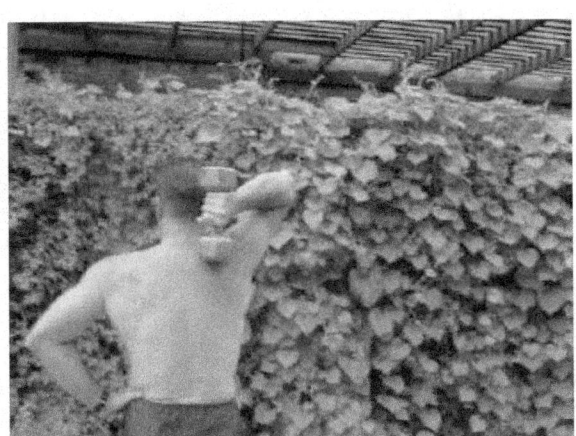
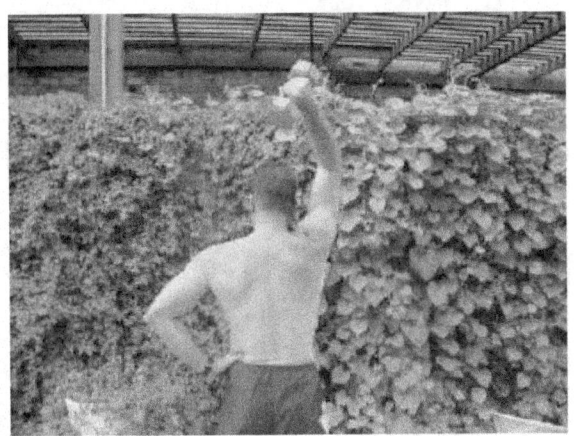

Stand with the feet about shoulder width apart lift the arms straight up in the air. Drop the weight directly behind the head and then push it up. Concentrate on the triceps. Be sure to keep the elbow straight.

DUMBELLS

concentration curls

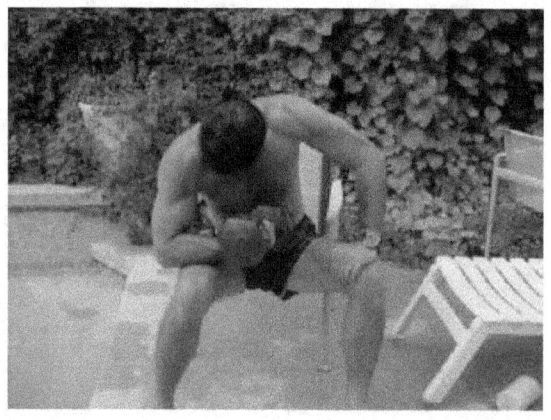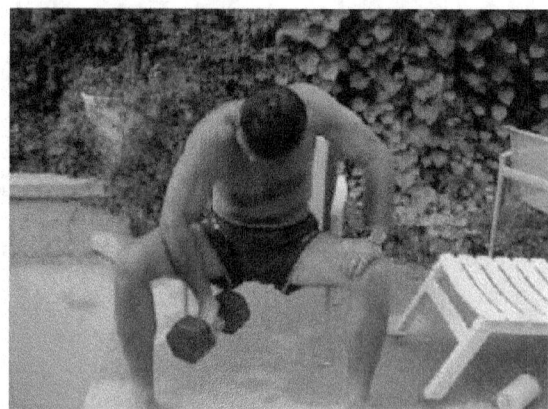

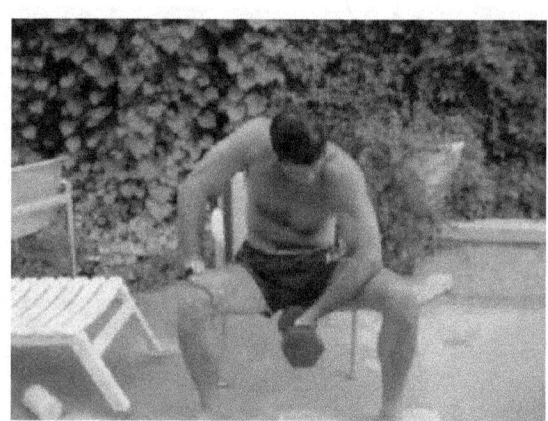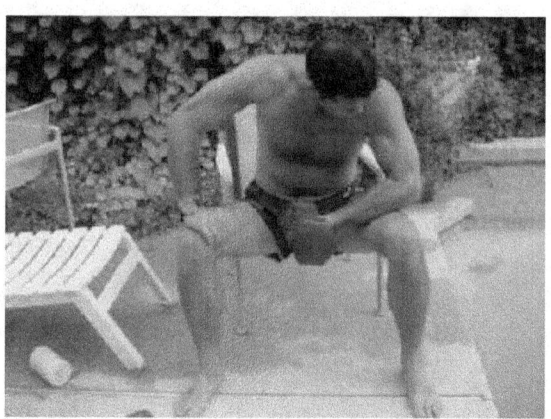

This is a concentration curl and really concentrates the muscles of the biceps. Sit in the chair and curl the weight up across the body. Keep the elbow on the knee..

Do 4 sets of 12 to 16 reps.

DUMBELLS

squats

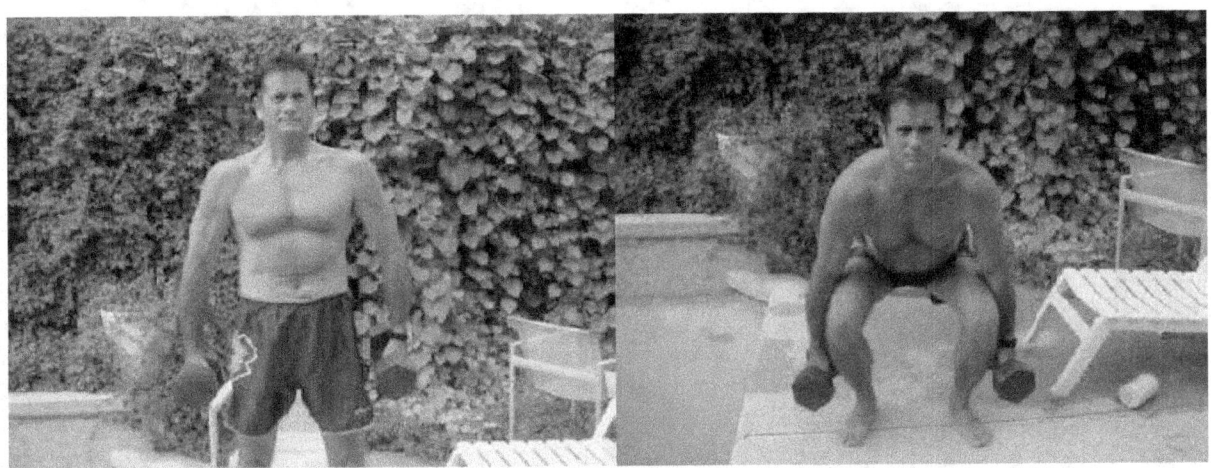

This is the only type of squat I recommend. It does not hurt the back or knees. Hold the weights in both hands and squat down, then back up.

Do 4 sets of 12 to 16 reps.

DUMBELLS

Walking with weights

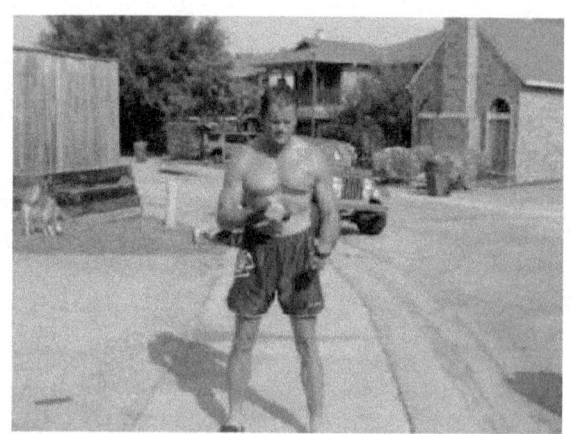 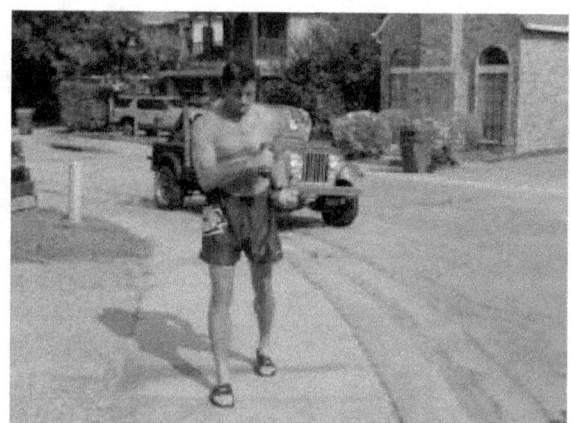

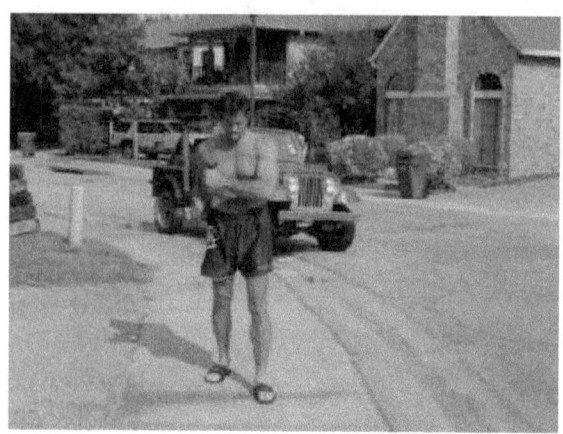 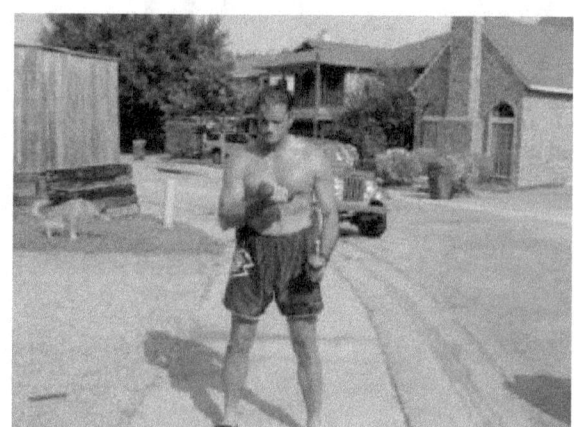

I never walk without my weights, even when playing golf. The weights give you twice the effect of regular walking. The walking helps tone your legs, butt and back, and the weights work your upper body.

I walk at least 1 mile to 3 miles, very quick. I do this at least 3 times a week, sometimes 5.

Sometimes I curl the weights across my body.
Alternating hands.

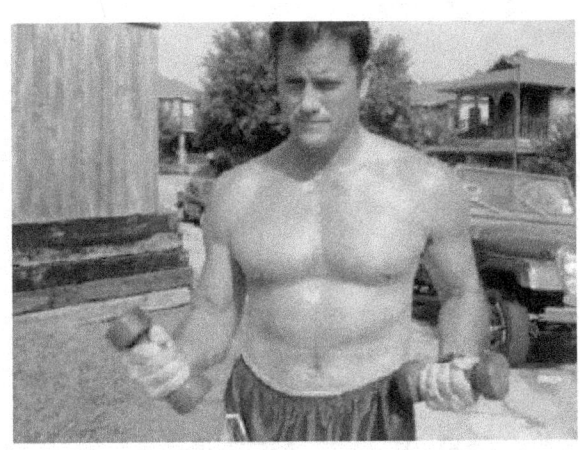 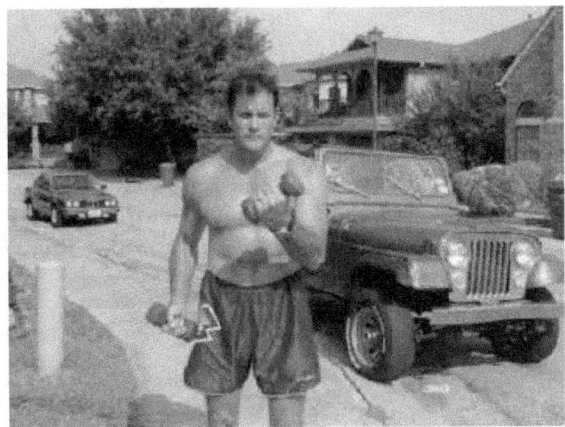

Sometimes I punch the weights in front of my
body. Twisting the wrist at the end of the punch.

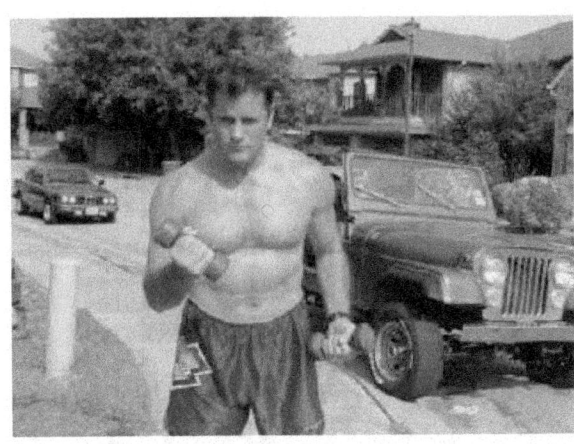 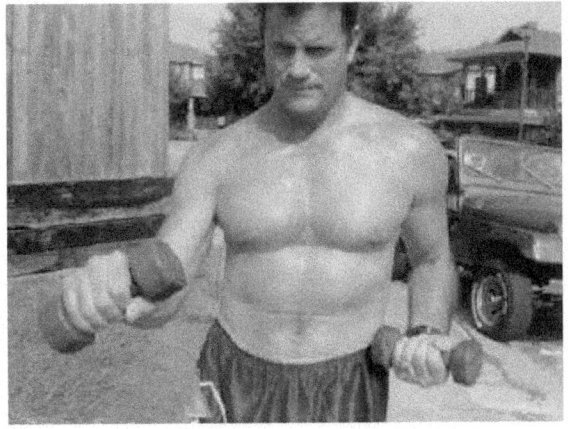

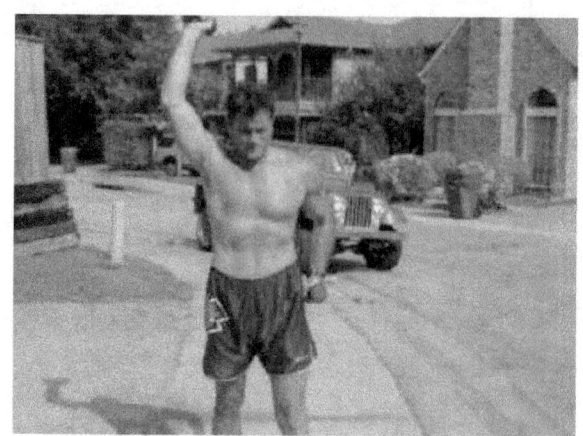

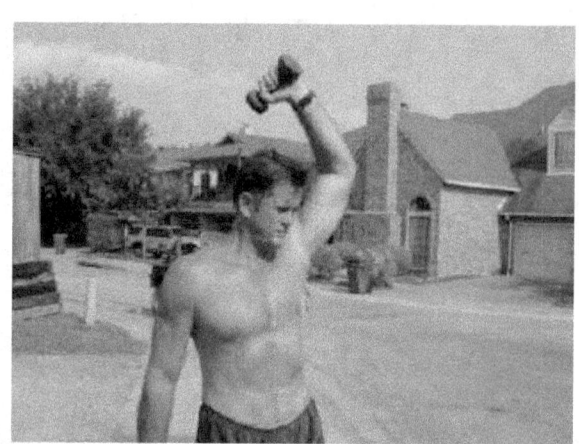

When my biceps get tired I
immediately go to triceps
extensions with alternating
arms.
I do this as many times as I
can, usually about ¼ a mile.

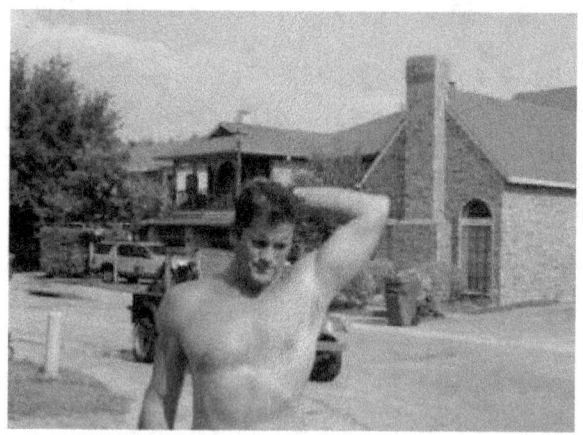

Building muscles without weights

chair triceps

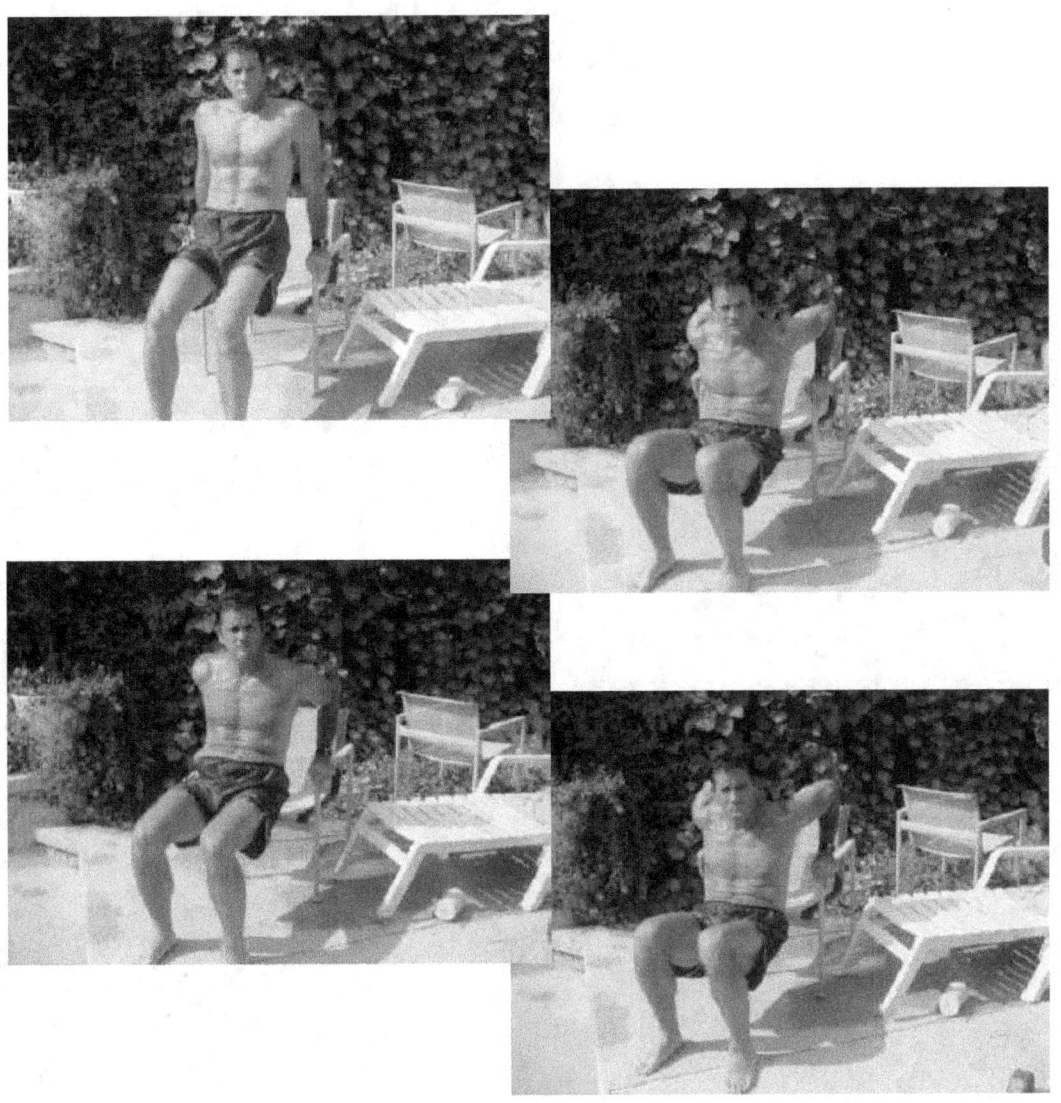

You can pump up the triceps by doing dips from a chair. It also works the chest. Hold the arms of the chair and dip down as low as you can. Concentrate on the triceps and chest.

I do 5 sets of 50 reps.

Building muscles without weights
Truck triceps

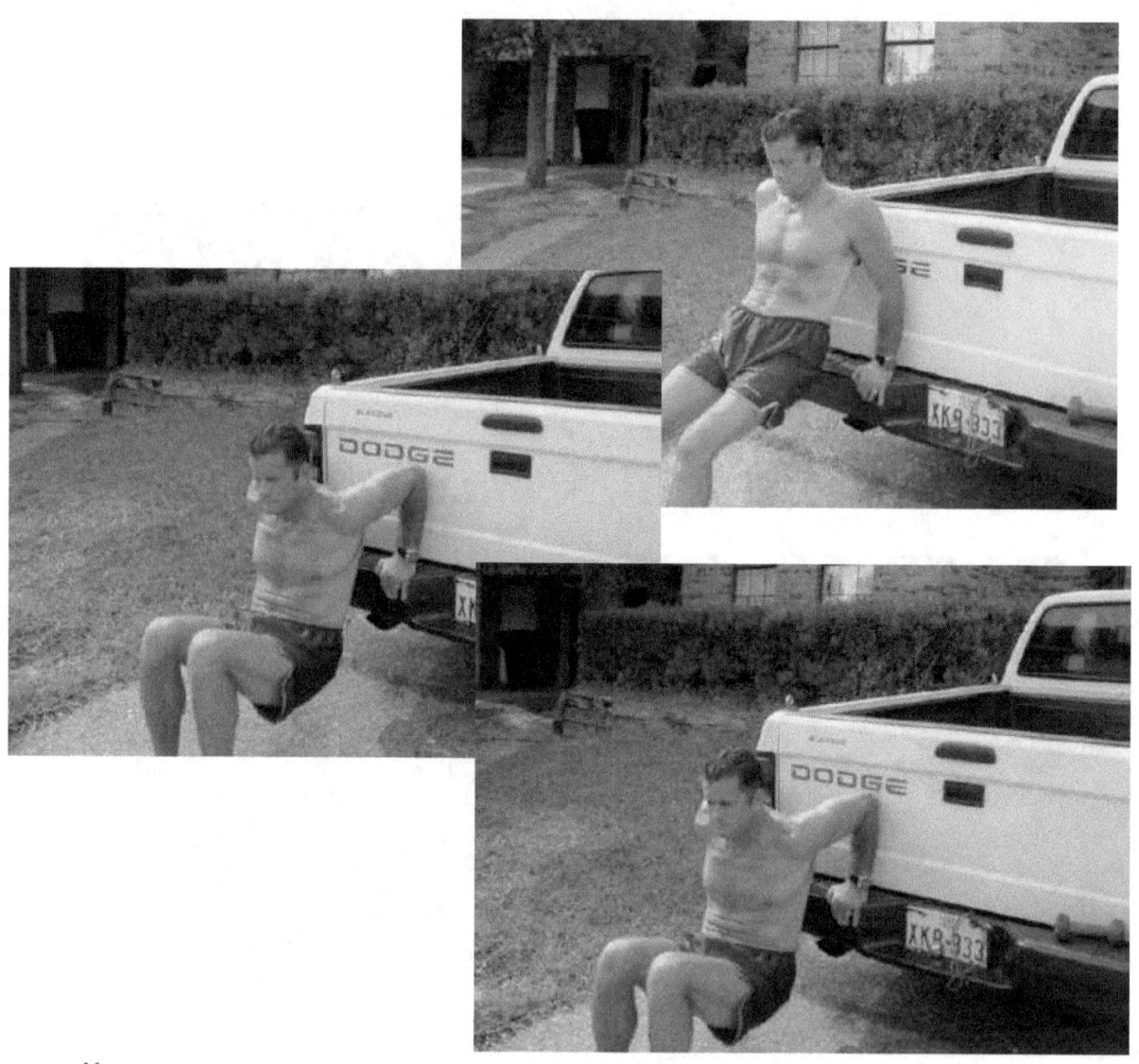

You can pump up the triceps by doing dips from the bumper of a truck, or car. It also works the chest. Hold the arms of the chair and dip down as low as you can. Concentrate on the triceps and chest.

I do 5 sets of 50 reps.

Building muscles without weights
Ground triceps

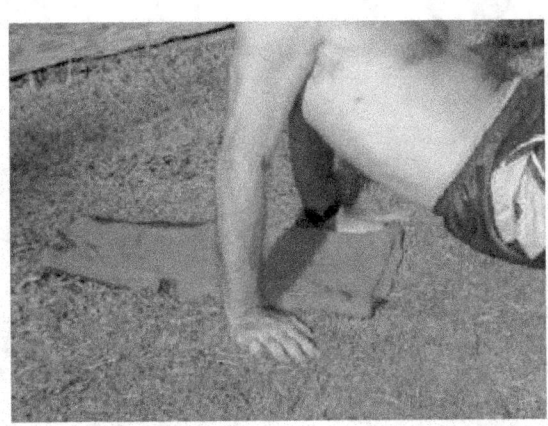

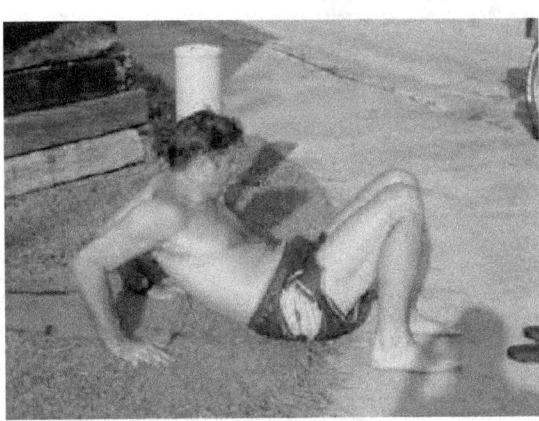
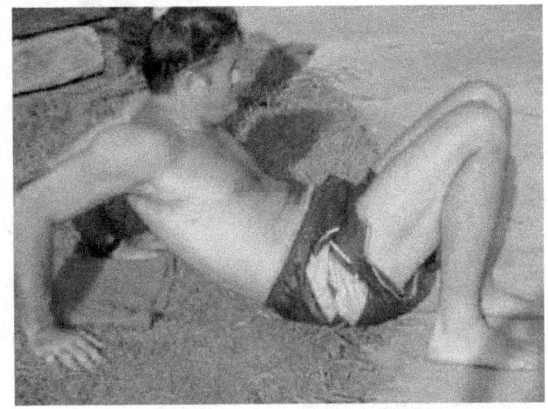

You can pump up the triceps on the ground without weights by lifting the body off the ground and dipping down to the middle. Concentrate on the triceps.

I do 5 sets of 25 reps.

Building muscles without weights

super push ups

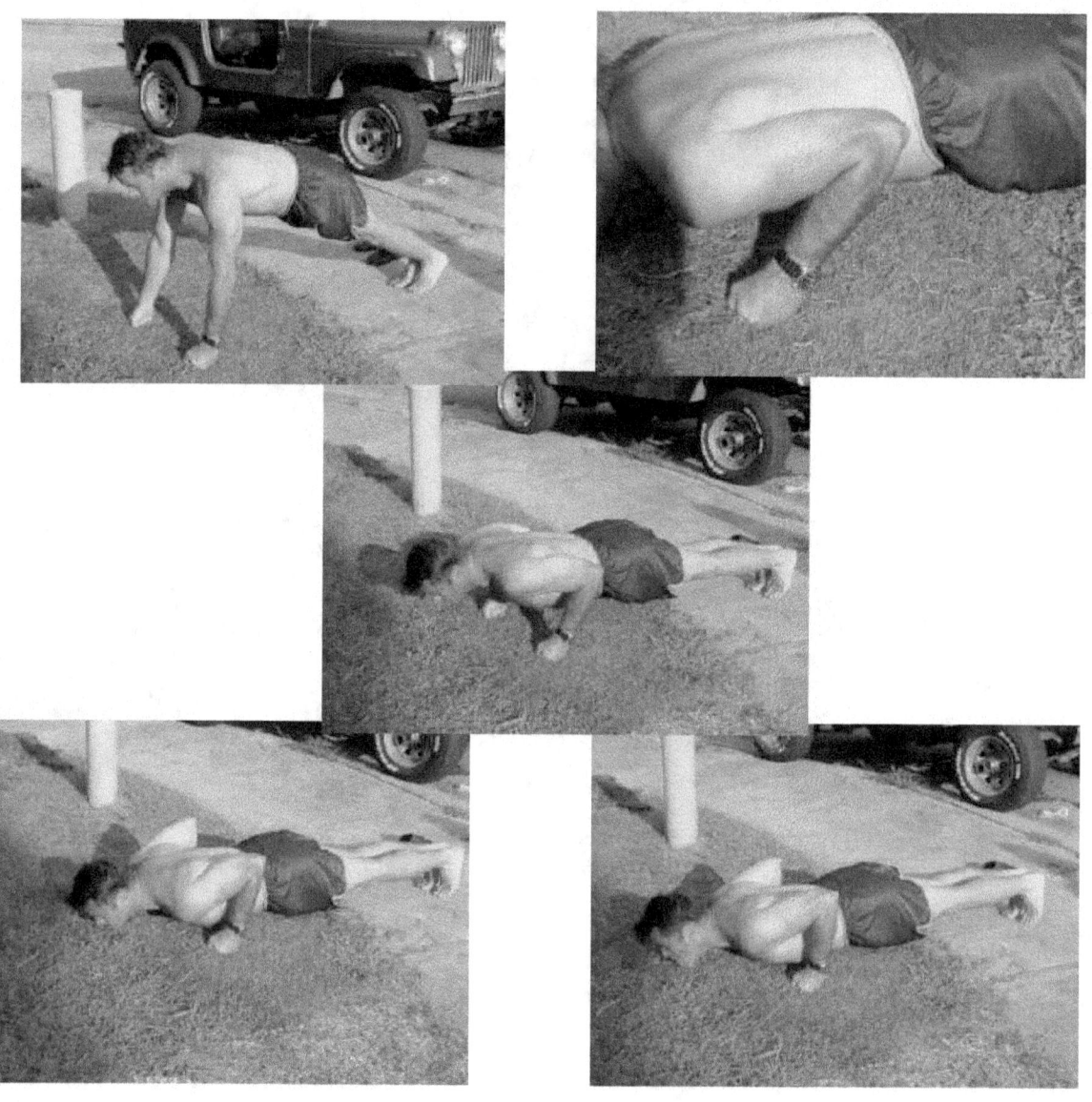

I do a modified push up where I do not come all the way up. I keep my arms fairly close to the body and go all the way down, but only up about 6 to 12 inches. This really pumps the chest, arms and shoulders.

I do sets of 100 to 150. I do 5 to 10 sets. For 500 to 1,000 push ups.

Building muscles without weights
super push ups 2

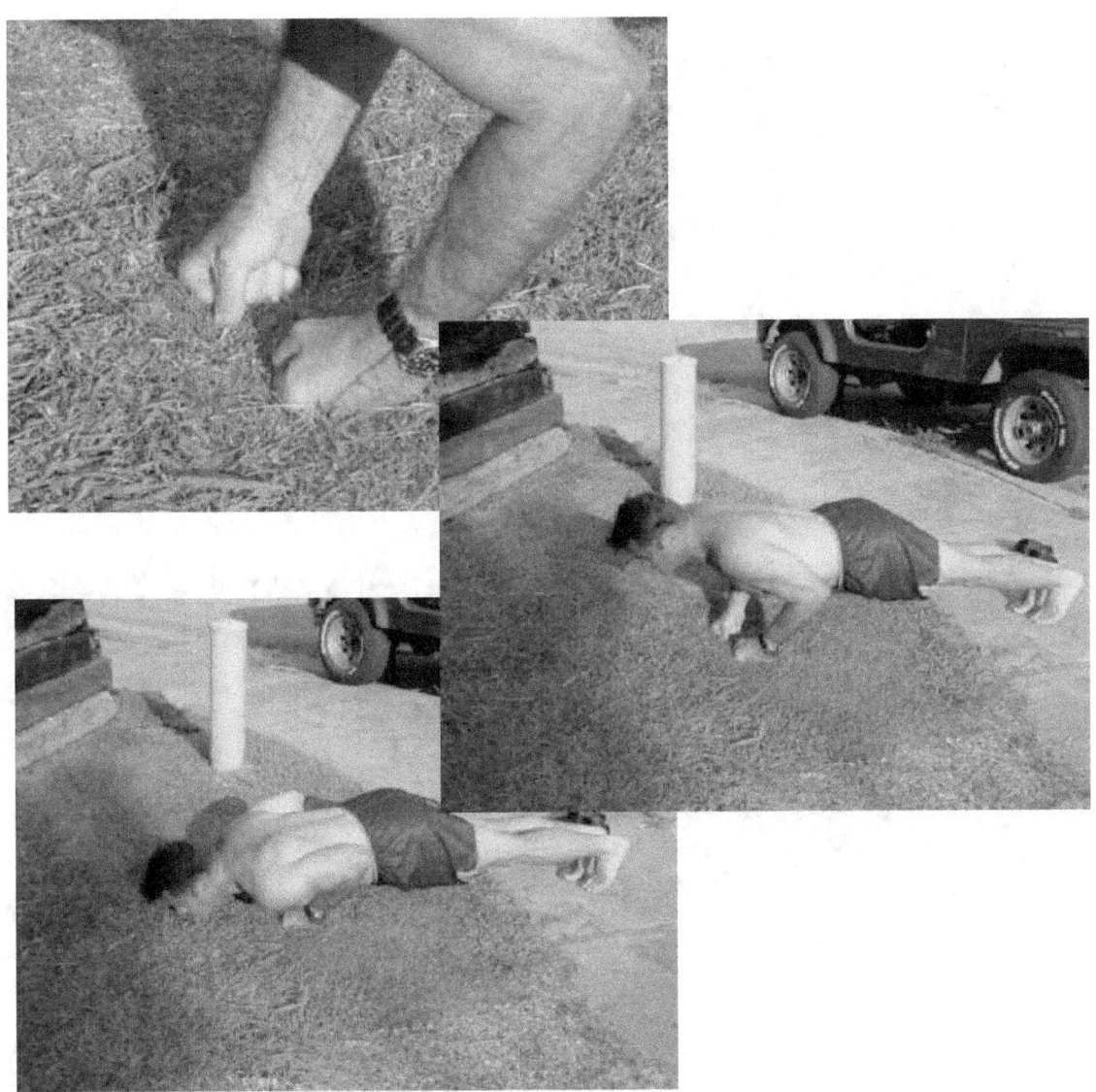

This is done the same way as super push ups, but with the arms held close together, to really work the inside of the chest. I go all the way down, but only up about 6 to 12 inches. This really pumps the chest, arms and shoulders.

I do sets of 50. I do 5 to 10 sets.

abdominals

Sits ups in a chair

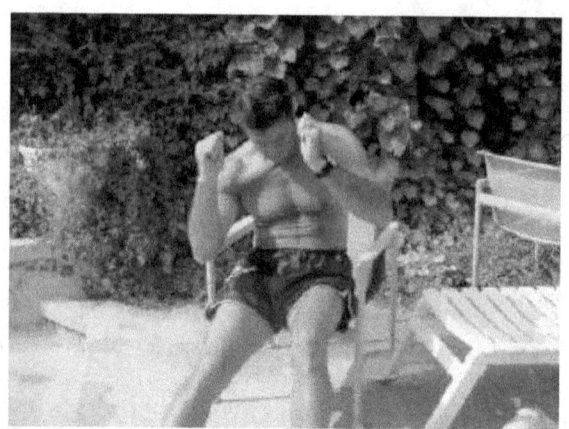 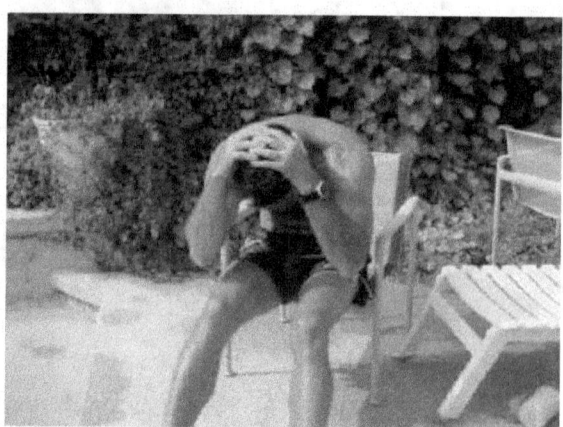

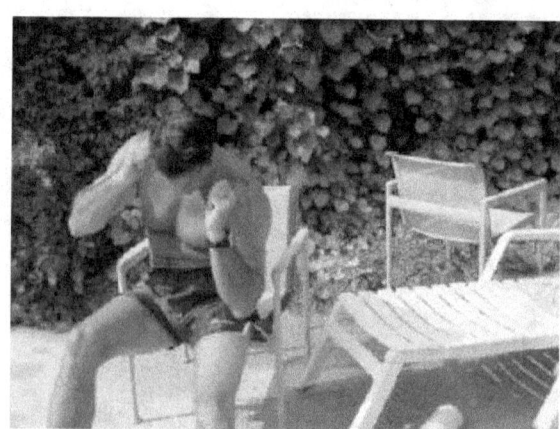 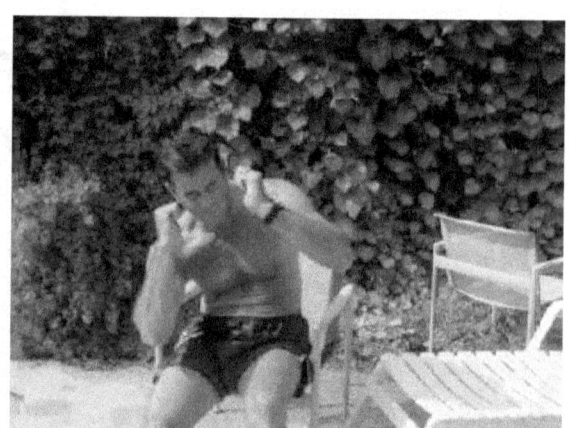

You heard me right. You can do sit ups from a chair and work the abs just as hard as if you were on the ground. You simply crunch your abs to the left and right and then down the middle. They are very effective and really work the abs.

I do a lot. I do sets of 50 to each side, and 50 to the middle. 4 sets.

abdominals

Sits ups

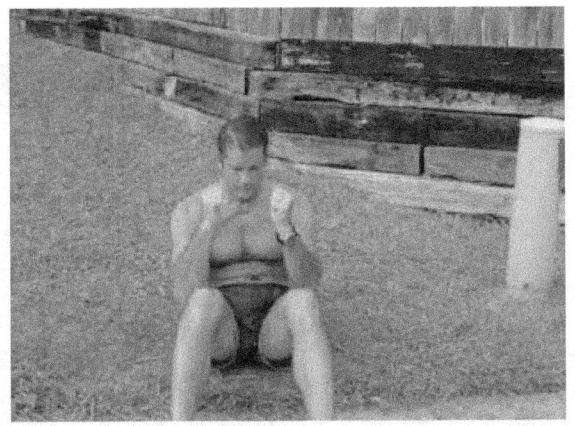 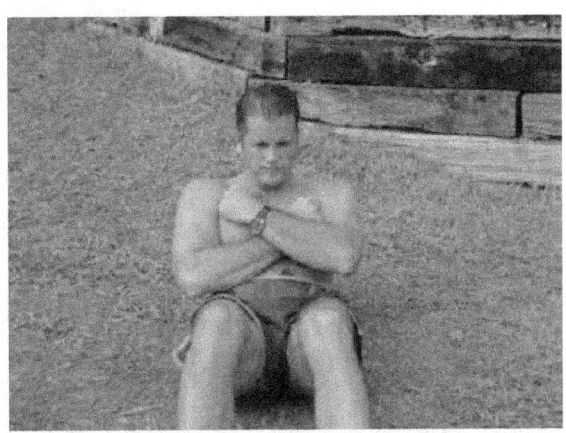

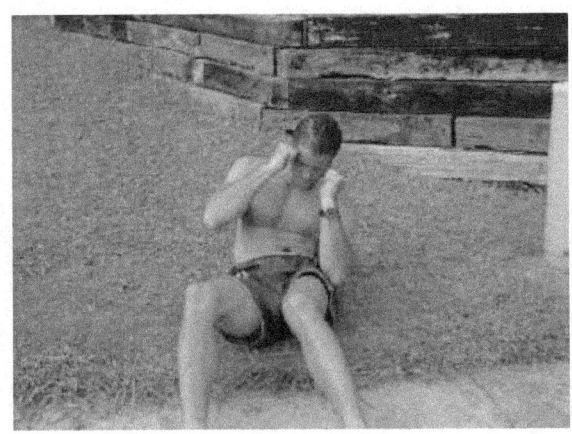 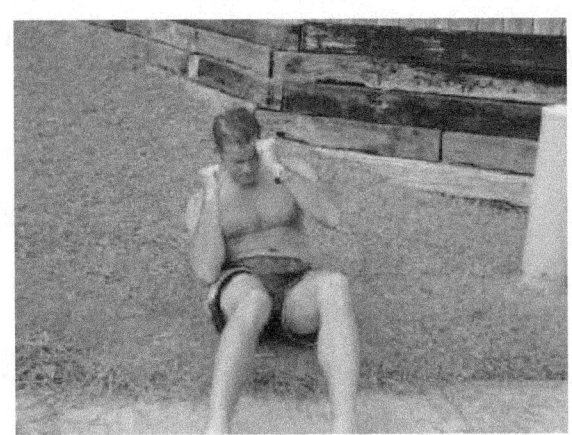

You can't do enough sits. I do hundreds a day, sometimes a thousand. I do them without my feet pushed against anything or under anything, and I lean to the right and left when I work, so I can work each side of the abs and the muscles that surround the

I never put the hands behind the head, and never go all the way back. When you go to down to the ground and lie flat you are resting, and when you start to come up you hurt your neck, and do not work your abs.

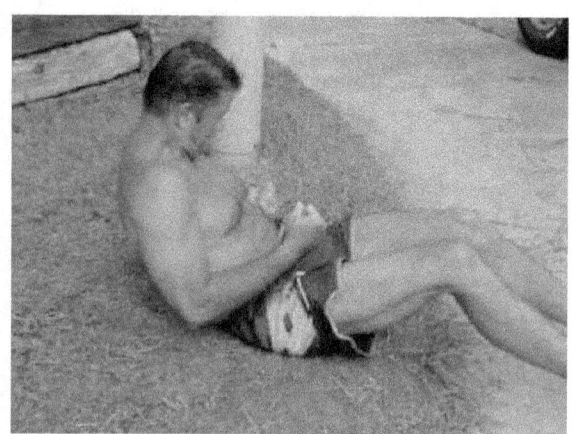 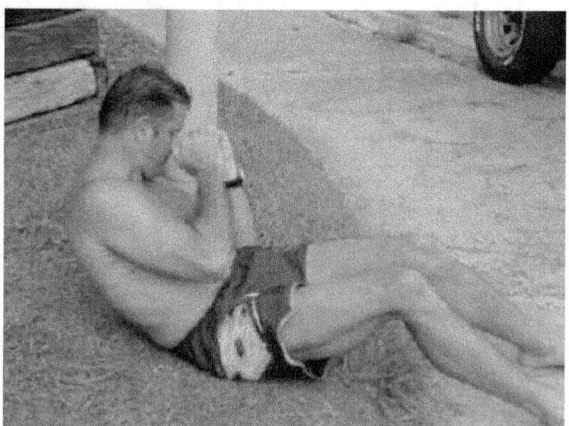

I always twist to the side and punch up to work my arms too.

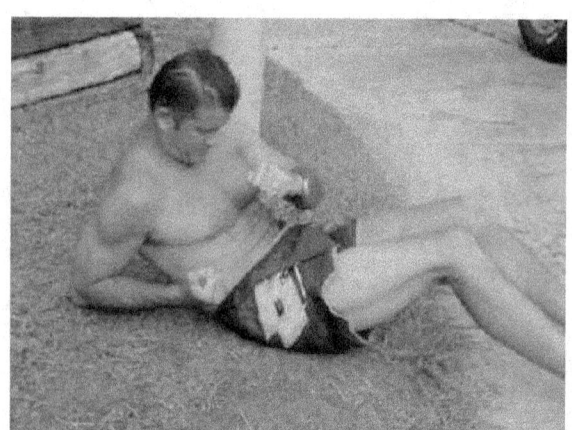 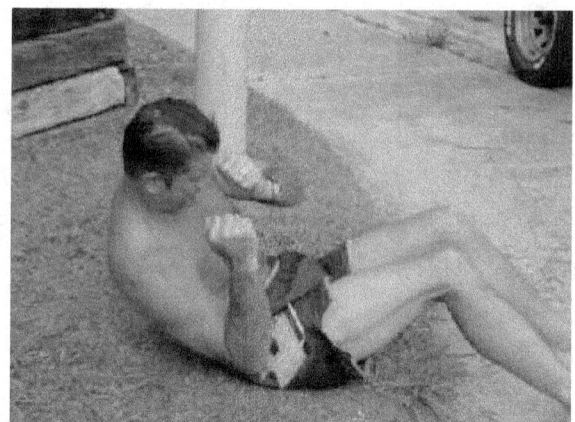

I do sets of 50 on each side and then 50 in the middle. For a total of 150, then I rest and do it again. This is one set. I do 5 sets for 750 sits ups.

Abdominal
crunches

Crunches are a modified sit up that tightens the abs but doesn't hurt the back. This time you put your hands behind the head and crunch up as far as you can, at least 6 inches off the ground.

I try to do 50 reps at a time in sets of 5.

You can also pull the legs into the arms To really concentrate the crunch.

Abdominal
Arms ups & v ups

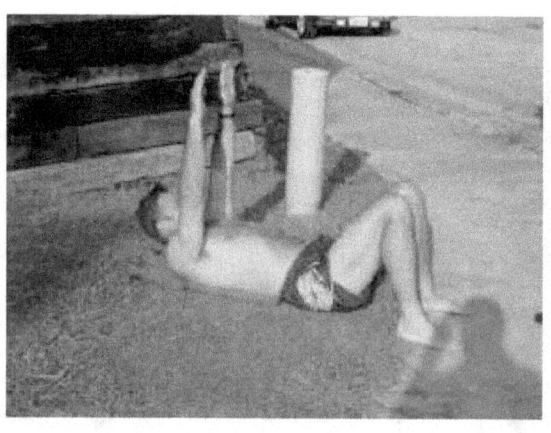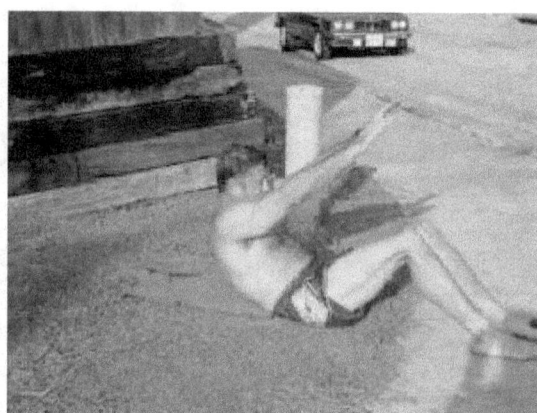

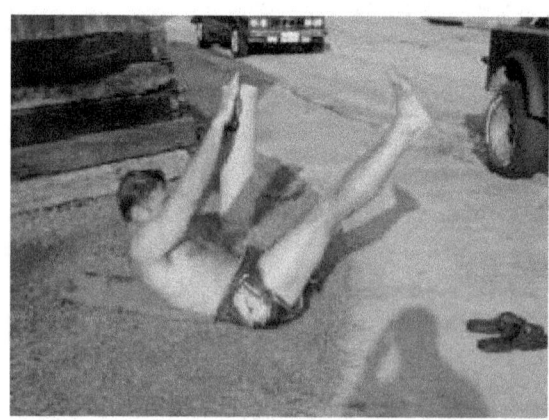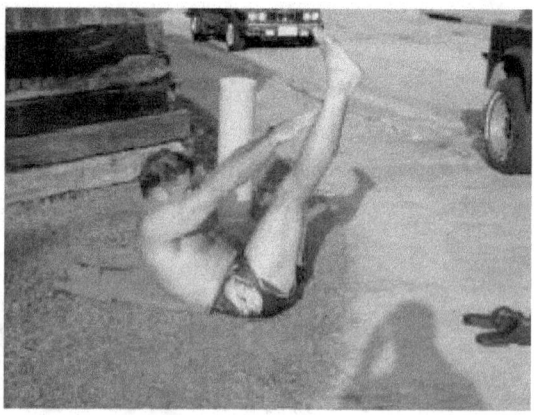

Hold the arms straight up and pull yourself off the ground. You can also pull the legs back and try to touch the toes as you lift the head towards the legs.

Do 3 sets to 25 reps.

Back strengthening

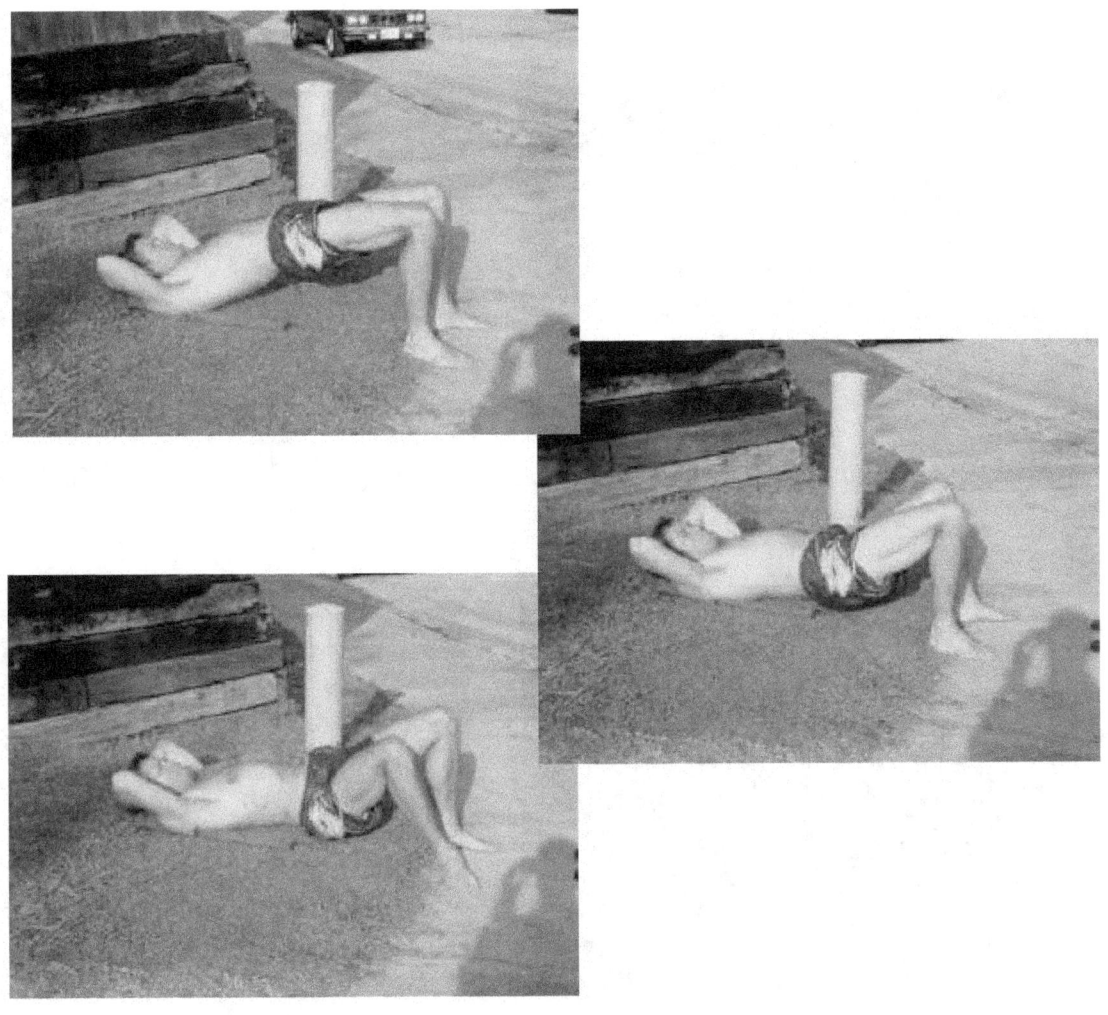

Lie on your back and put your hands behind your head. Lift the
butt off the ground and up as high as you can. Drop your weight
down first to the right side then to your left side.
This will help strengthen you lower back.
Do 4 sets of 12 to 16 reps.

abdominals
Leg lifts in a chair

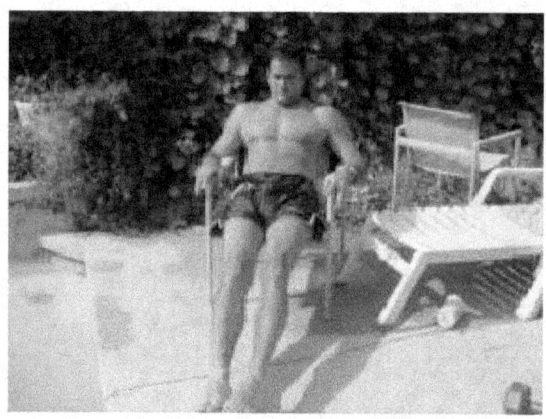 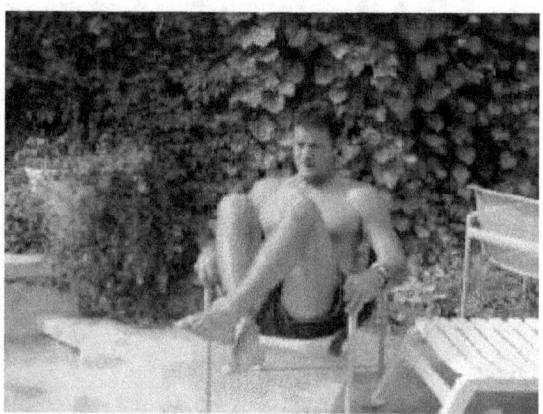

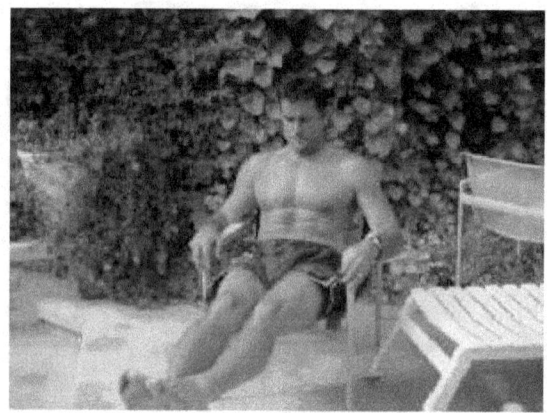 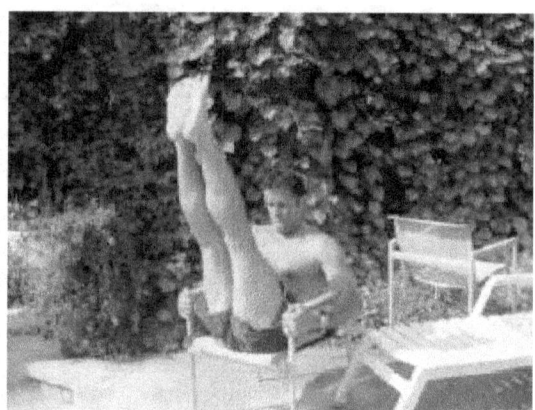

You can really work the lower abs by doing leg lifts in a chair. You can concentrate on the legs and use the chair for support and not hurt the back. Keep the legs straight and lift them straight up.

For a variation you can curl them straight back.

I do a lot. I do sets of 50 to each side, and 50 to the middle. 4 sets.

Abdominal
Leg lifts

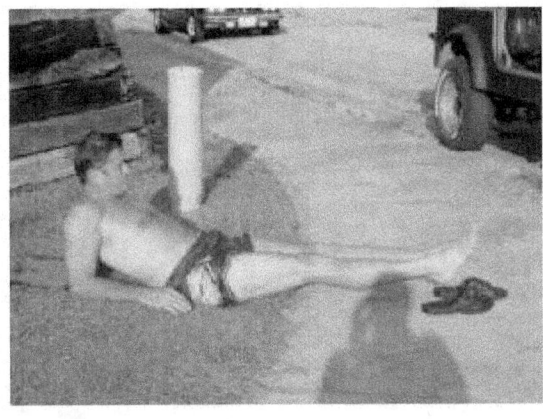 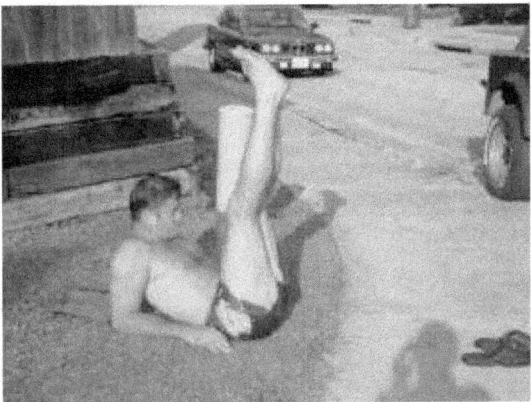

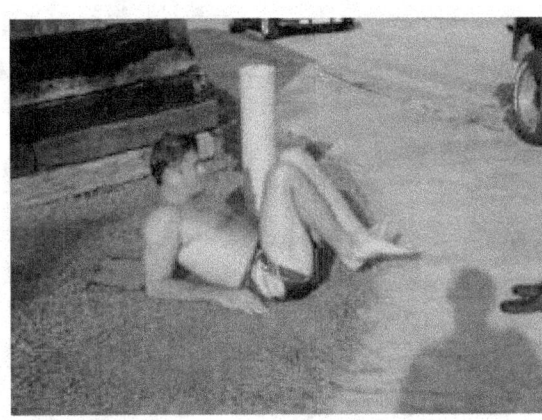 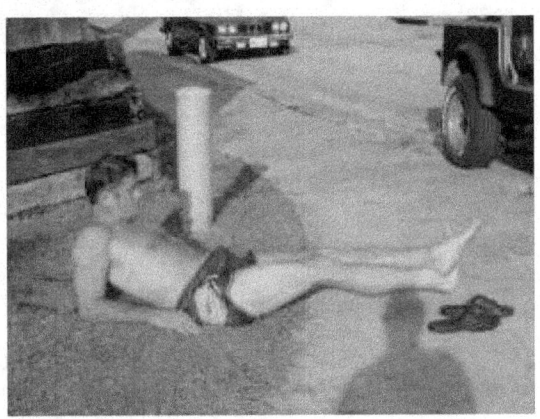

Leg Litts are important for several reasons. They work the lower abs and the help strengthen the back, as well as the knees. Keep the toes pointed and the legs straight. You can lift them straight up or curl them back into the abs.

I do a lot. I try to do them for 3 minutes without stopping. I can usually do 180 or more in the 3 minutes.

Abdominal
Side bends

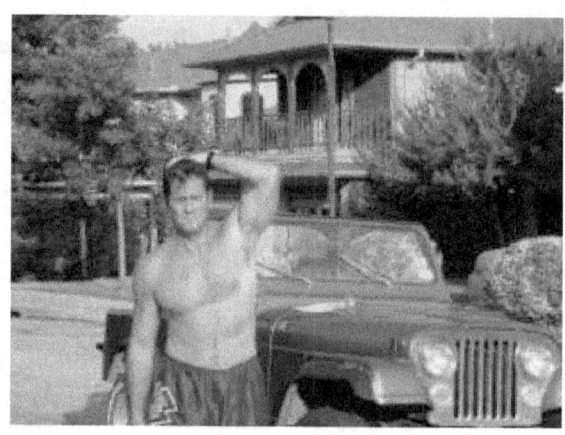

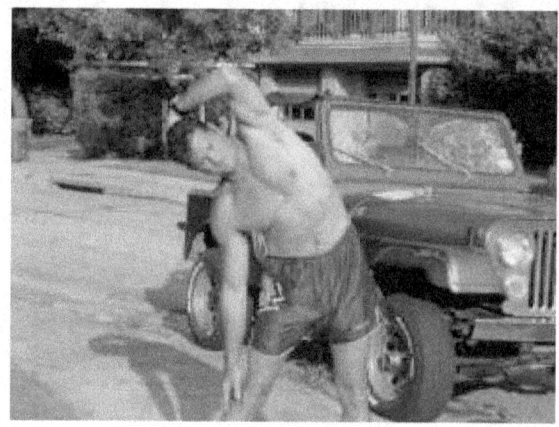 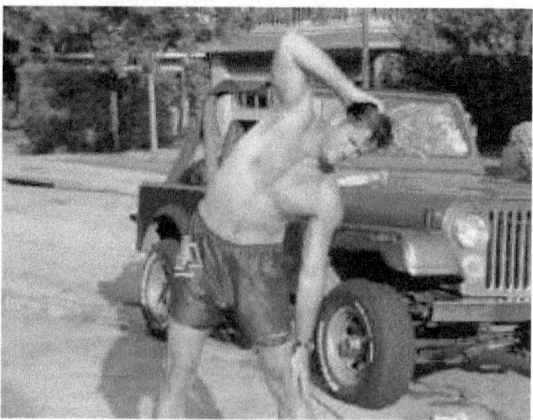

Side bens really work to get rid of that love muscle or bulge around the waist. Hold one hand on the head and lean to the right and left side as far as you can.

Do 3 sets to 25 reps each side.

Building muscles without weights
Circular Breathing

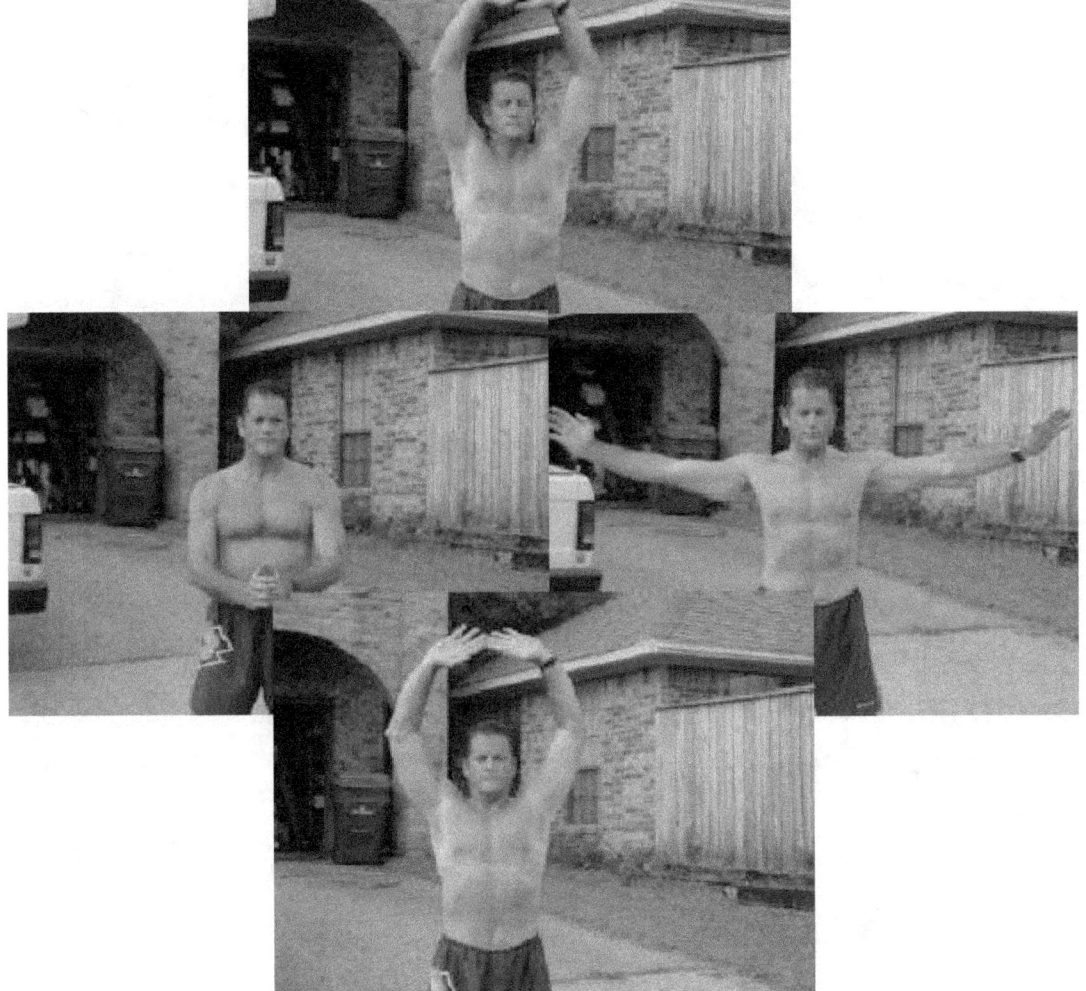

Circular Breathing is the fastest way to recover your breath after hard exercise. It allows for the full expansion of your lungs and full removal of air that is bad.

Hold the arms above the head and while breathing in make a large circle with your arms until they touch in front. Then breath out making the same large circle.

Do about 5 times to recover your breath after hard exercise.

Building muscles without weights
4 way Breathing

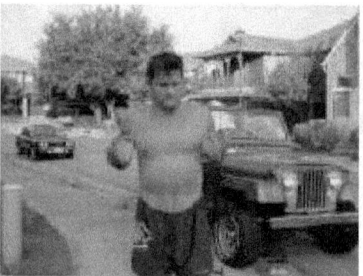

4 Way Breathing is a way to tighten all the muscles of the body, especially the abs and back. It is an extreme isometric exercise and forces you to concentrate on getting all the air out of your body and tightening the muscles.

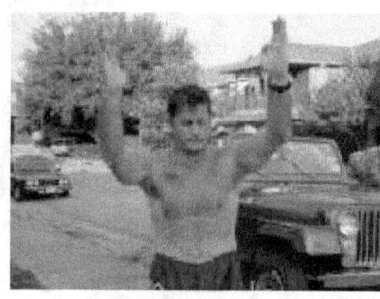

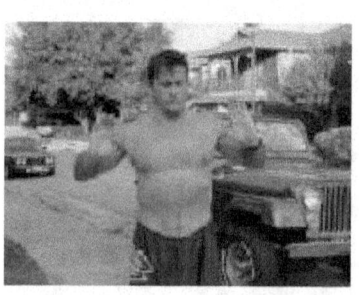

Start with the arms in front of the body and slowly move the arms straight up, tightening every muscle and concentrating on removing all the air from the stomach.

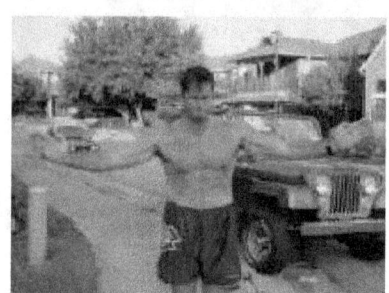

Return the arms, and now go out to the side, then to the front and finally straight down.

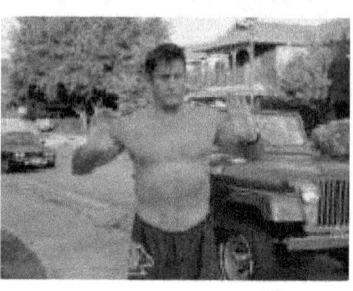

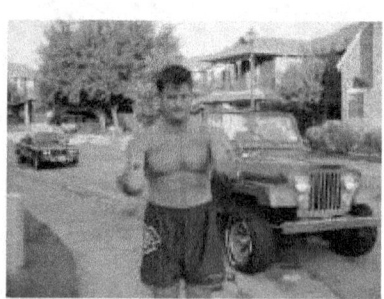

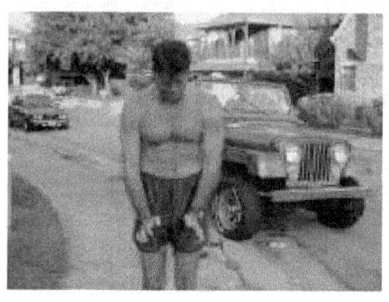

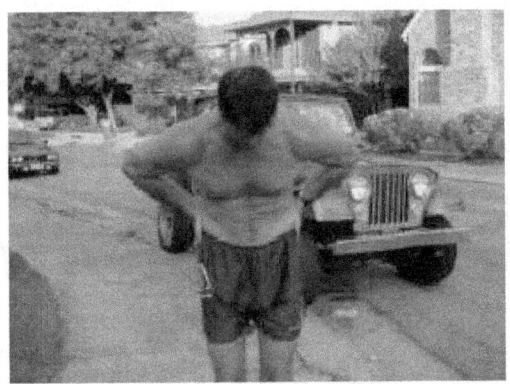

After you have done the 4 way breathing holds the arms to the sides of the body and really tighten and squeeze the stomach muscles, breathing out, and squeezing very very hard to clear all the air from the stomach.

This exercise helps develop KI and I test my KI by punching myself in the stomach very hard. You do not have to punch yourself, unless you want to.

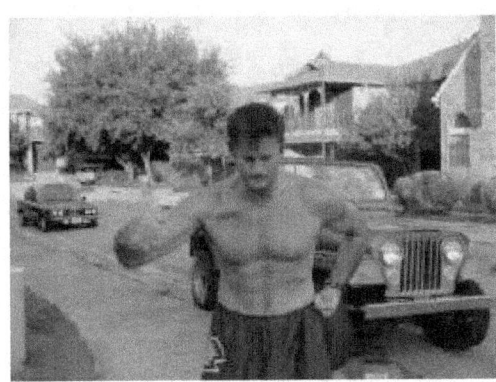 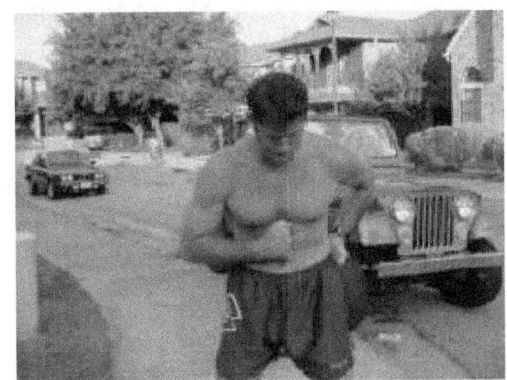

Building muscles without weights
Isometric Breathing

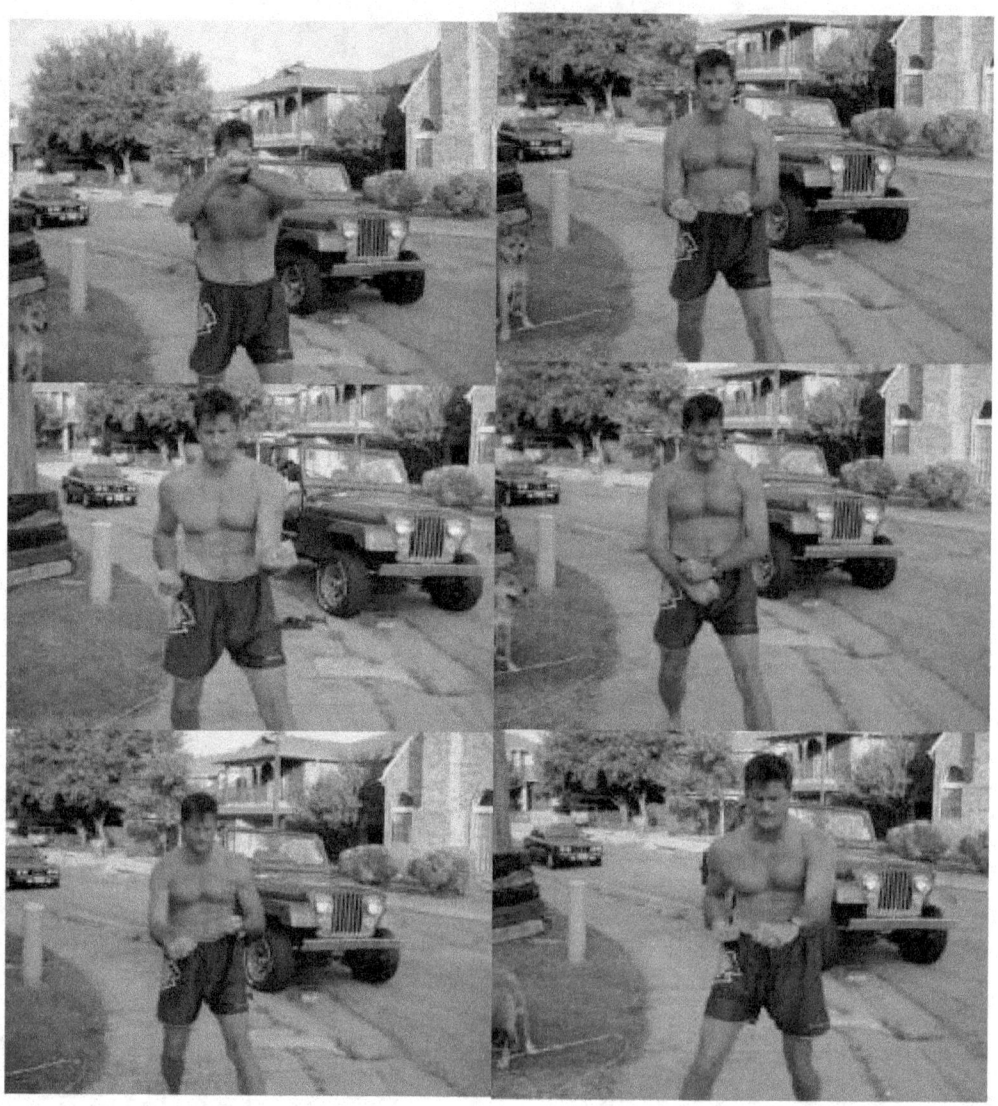

Isometric breathing is an important concept and exercise to understand. It is a fundamental exercise of the martial arts. It is in all forms and called "sonchin" in my style of karate. It is very simple to explain, but very difficult to master.

Unlike tai chi, which is breathing very soft and moving very fluid. Isometric breathing is breathing very forcefully and moving very hard, but slow.

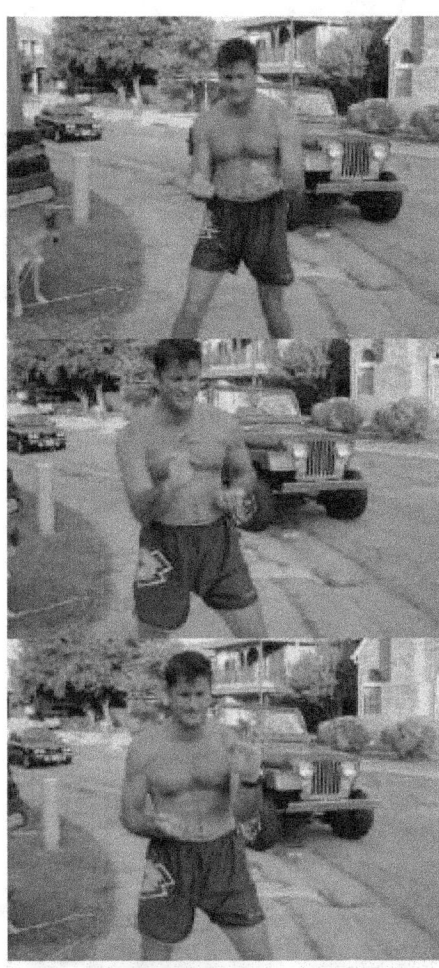

To do the exercises you must first start with the body very tight and concentrate on the breath.

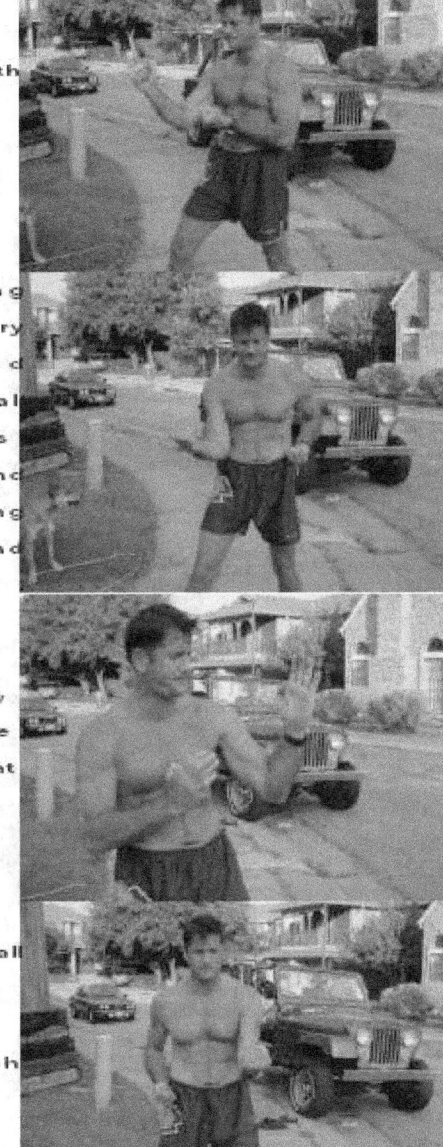

Now breathing out move very slowly and forcefully in all directions Pushing one hand out and pulling the other hand back

You can punch across the body, to the side of the body, to the front of the body, down and even up.

You must force all the air out, and tighten all the muscles on each punching or pushing drill.

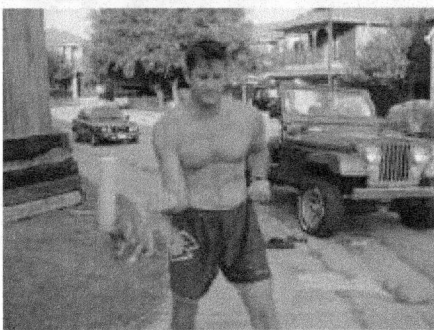

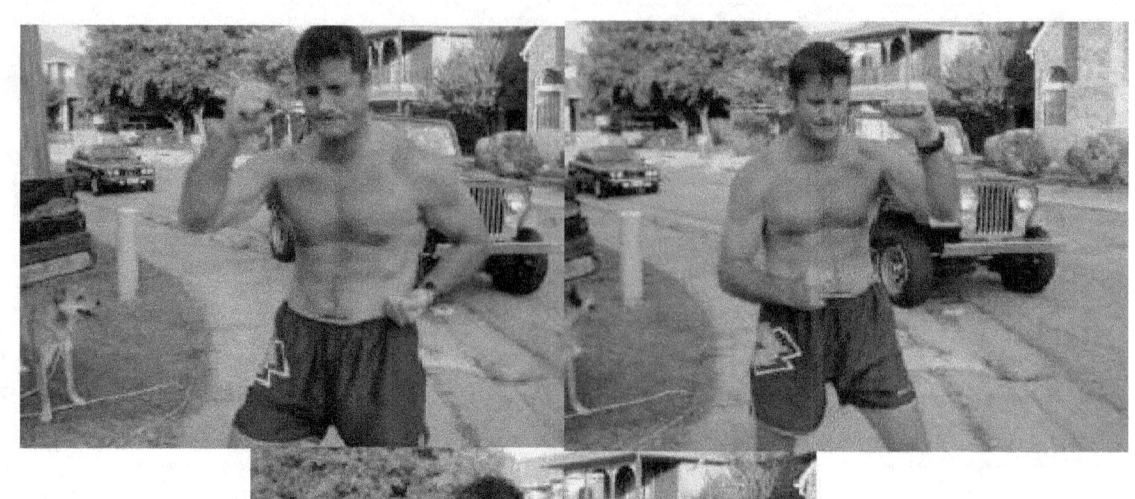

The key to doing the exercises right is to force the air out and tighten the muscles. When you push or punch out with one hand, you pull back with the other hand.

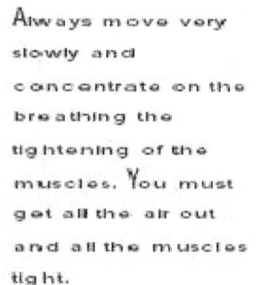

Always move very slowly and concentrate on the breathing the tightening of the muscles. You must get all the air out and all the muscles tight.

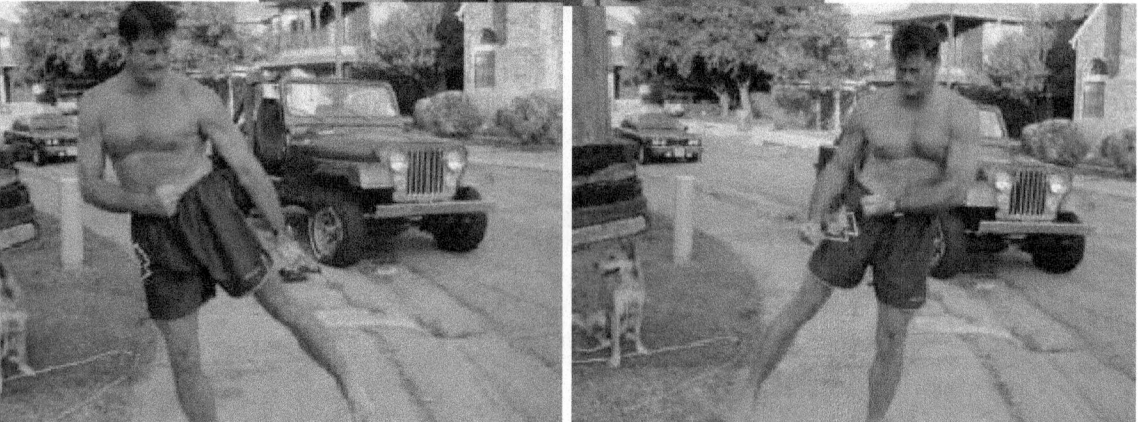

You can also push out the legs in a low kick and breath out very hard and tighten the muscles very hard. Remember to breath slowly, move slowly and concentrate.

There is a force in your body that creates incredible power. This force when used will enable the body to perform almost superhuman feats. It will allow you to with stand extremes of weather. **To take full power strikes to your body and receive absolutely no injury, even a bruise from a blow that would Kill a normal person.** This is called HARD KI. To control your mental focus for hours, days. To develop inner strength an power you can only imagine. This is the power of KI, sometimes called Chi. And this is a power you can learn to develop and use at will for your entire life.

KI is a concept that is unfamiliar to many Americans, but understood and practiced by most Orientals. The concept of KI is 3000 years old and was developed by the Buddhist monks of the Sholan Monastery of China.

Many teachers only teach parts of the power of KI and the students learning do not fully develop their KI. We will be learning to develop and use Hard KI. To fully understand how to use and develop your KI you must understand that KI is really 3 elements in one. When all 3 elements are fully developed, you have full Hard KI. Hard KI uses all 3 elements to create its full power, and if you don't use all 3 elements, and develop each fully and independently you will not develop your full Hard KI.

So what are the 3 elements of Hard KI.

(1) Muscle control. The instantaneous tightening of specific muscles at the time of impact, and the development of essential muscles necessary to withstand various kicks and punches.

(2) Breath control. The science of controlling the rate and the movement of the breath. The ability to forcibly, at the instant of impact remove all breath from your body to allow the muscles full contraction of the muscles, and to strengthen the concentration of the mind.

(3) Mind control. The specific concentration of mental powers and focus of the mind. The total concentration of your mental processes towards a specific goal, area,

or muscle. The ability for complete and total mental focus so that nothing can distract the minds power.

Separately these three forces constitute functions, activities and parts of your body, but when they are joined together and united at a specific time towards a specifid purpose they take on a single identity of a new force, called KI. KI can be used to protect you from receiving an injury associated with a punch or a blow, to increase your determination, give you courage, improve your skills, add to your strength, develop your concentration to extreme levels.

Why does KI work? It works because you are using all the powers available in your body to prevent an injury, not just your muscle. Too many people think that muscle alone can prevent an injury from a blow. But examples in ordinary life prove the fallacy of this belief. Your leg is all muscle and if someone were to hit you in the leg very hard, you would at the least get a bruise, perhaps a charley horse, or a muscle injury. That is because it is actually too much muscle and as such cannot give any with the blow. It is like a tree that got covered with snow and finally the weight of the snow breaks the tree down, while a smaller more flexible tree can bend and touch the ground and not break. Your leg has all muscle and no give, so a hard blow breaks the muscle tissue and causes the bruises. It is also possible to make the stomach very hard by the use of sit ups and leg ups and if you tighten it you can let someone punch you in the stomach. However take a deep breath of air into your stomach and let someone hit you in the stomach. A very slight blow would cause a significant amount of damage because the air acts like a balloon and explodes or pops in the stomach area causing internal damage. Let us suppose that you can take a punch in the stomach and you have let most of your air out. But before you are ready for the punch, someone comes up and asks you a question, momentarily distracting your attention, and you are suddenly hit. Needless to say, you could be very seriously injured because your mind was not prepared for the blow. So you can see it takes all three elements to protect the body from the effects of getting hit.

First you must have adequate muscle and muscle control so that your muscles are strong and can react and tighten at your will. You must be able to tighten and contract the muscles at the exact time and point of the impact of the blow.

Secondly, you must have some breath control and be breathing out, or moving your breath away from the area getting hit. You can not hold your breath and have Hard KI. You can not breath too fast, or too shallow, or forget to breath at all.

Third, you must have your mind controlled and focused to be aware that you are getting hit and to concentrate the muscles and breath simultaneously at the point of impact. Your mind must be at a constant ready and react immediately and precisely to the attack.

With these three factors working for you, **your KI is said to be "flowing"** and you are able to resist blows that would cripple normal people. Yet you too are normal. It is just that you have been able to, by practice, and the use of positive reinforcement and progressive training, apply your muscle, breath and mind to such states that you are able to focus them simultaneously and instantaneously to the area of impact when you see a blow about to occur.

We have already been shown exercises to strengthen the muscles, and to begin to concentrate and focus the mind. Now we will begin to do exercises to strengthen ones breath control. So we begin our development of KI by learn to control the breath.

CONTROLLING THE BREATH.

The first step in controlling the breath is to become aware of it as a force, and to use it to store (KI)in your body. Note: your KI is stored about 2 inches below your navel. This is your point of reference for KI in your body. And this point or KI center serves as a concentration and focus point for the mind when developing control of the breath and understanding of KI.

Stomach Breathing or KI Storing

Stomach Breathing: The purpose of this exercise is to store your KI in your body. What you should be thinking when you are doing this exercise is that you are storing KI power in your body and this power will be used to prevent your injuries. While you are practicing the breathing, keep thinking in your mind that you are storing KI power in your body.

Breath out thru the mouth and concentrate on storing the KI in your KI center, about 2 inches below the navel.

KI (Muscle, Breath & Mind Control)

Stand with the feet wide, arms by the side, hands
clinched and breath deeply into the stomach thru
the nose.

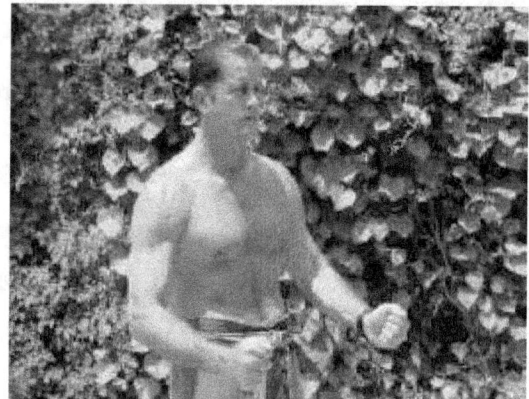

Stand with the feet shoulder width apart
with the arms by the side and the hands
closed into fists. Keep the mouth shut and
breathe through the nose. Keep the back
straight and the neck and heart in a straight
line. Begin to breathe in slowly but instead
of filling your chest with air, breathe into
the stomach, filling it with air. Hold it a
few seconds and begin to breathe out slowly, pulling in on the stomach gently as
you breathe out. Hold it a few seconds and repeat the exercise. Do this exercise for
2 minutes, all the time concentrating on the KI being stored. If you lose your
concentration, stop the exercise. This exercise only works when you believe and
concentrate on the fact that you are storing a power and when you keep the mind
concentrated on your breathing. You are doing this exercise both to control your
breath and to practice mind focus or concentration. Do this every day for at least 3
months, and then at least twice a week after you have developed your KI
sufficiently to receive very hard blows without injury.

Isotonic Breathing:

The purpose of this exercise is to begin to learn how to get all of the air out of the
body, especially the stomach area, by the concentration of the mind and the
tightening of the muscles to help to squeeze the air out. This is a 5 part exercise
and should be performed immediately after the stomach breathing, or KI storing
exercise.

1. Place the feet together, and keep the back straight.

2. Slowly begin to raise the arms straight up above the head to a full extension.

3. While raising the arms straight up, begin to let the air out of the stomach and
chest and as you get to the top begin to tighten the muscles of the entire body to
squeeze every last drop of air out of the stomach, and from the chest.

4. Hold this position for 3 seconds and really concentrate to get every drop of air out of the body, as well as concentrating on tightening every muscle of the body to help squeeze the air out.

5. Bring the arms back to the level of the shoulders and slowly begin to push the arms out straight to the sides.

6. While pushing the arms out to the sides, concentrate to tighten every muscle of the body and to get every ounce of air out of the body.

7. Hold your full extension for 3 seconds and really concentrate on getting all the air out of the body and on the tightening of all muscles of the body.

8. Slowly bring the arms back to the level of the shoulders and now begin to push them out straight ahead of the body.

9. While pushing the arms straight ahead concentrate to tighten all the muscles and to squeeze all the air out of the body.

10. Hold your full extension straight ahead for 3 seconds and really concentrate. Now slowly return the arms to the shoulders.

11. Slowly push the arms straight down in front of the body.

12. Concentrate all the muscles to squeeze the air out.

13. Hold your full downward extension for 3 seconds and then slowly bring the arms up to the chest.

14. Open the legs, tighten the fists and slightly lean over and concentrate on tightening all the muscles of the stomach as hard as you can. Try to crunch down the stomach muscles and squeeze the stomach muscles together (like an accordion). Do this around 15 seconds until you really begin to feel all the muscles of the stomach tightening. These exercises are excellent for learning to get the air out of the body, especially out of the stomach area. It helps one to practice mind control and concentration techniques
plus strengthens the muscles through isometric contraction.

Perform this exercise daily for at least 3 months until you have begun to be able to let someone hit you very hard in the solar plexus area and the ribs. Then you may practice it 2 to 3 times a week.

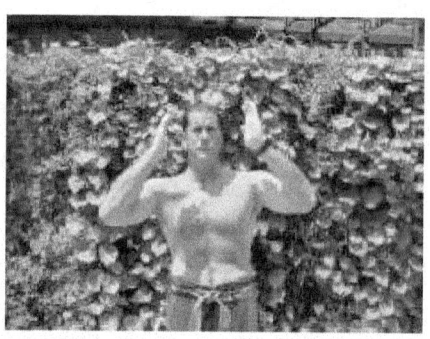

Hold the arms in front of the body before each push.

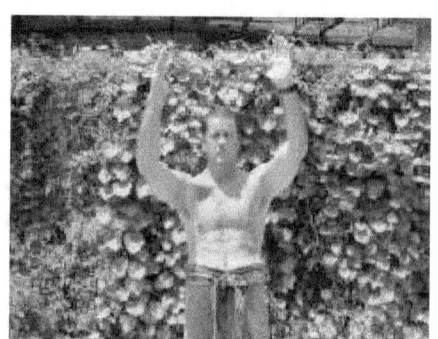

Push the arms straight up, tightening every muscle and forcing all air out of the body

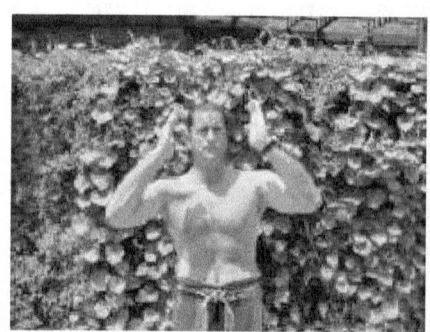

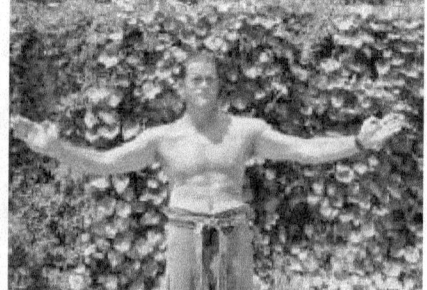

Return to the center and push the arms straight to the sides.

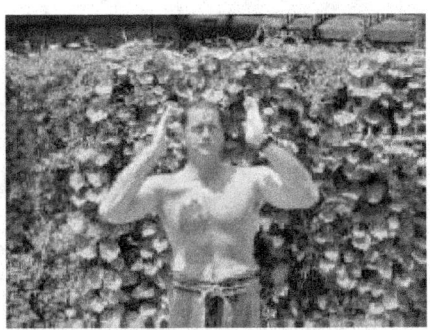 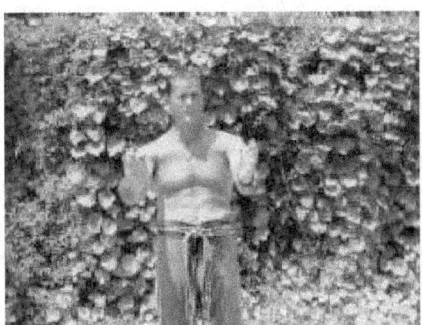

Return to the center and push the arms straight ahead.

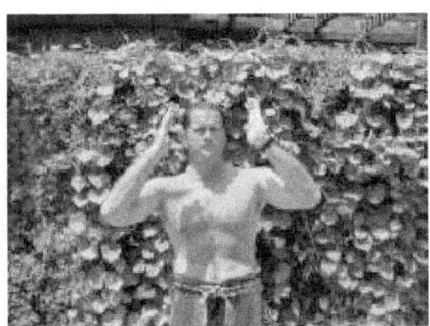 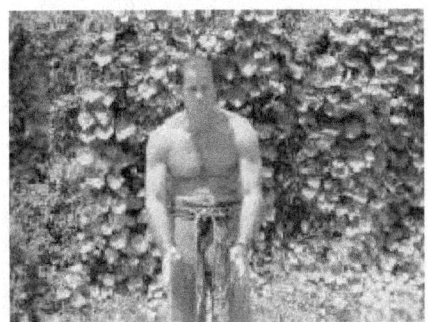

Return to the center and push the arms straight down.

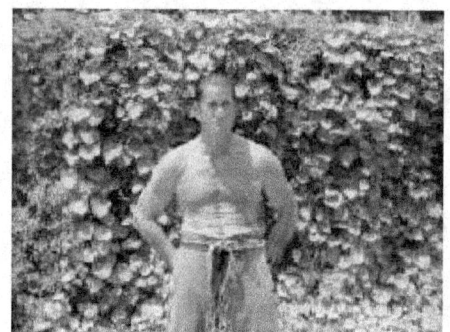 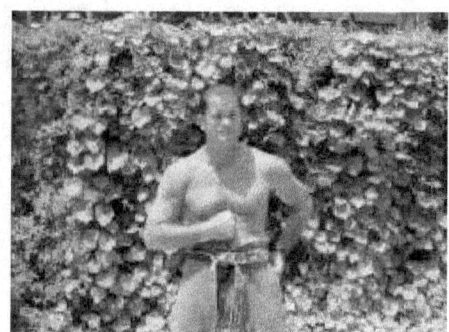

**Tighten all the muscles of the body, and force all the air out.
You may test that air being out of your body by punching
yourself in the stomach very hard.**

BEGINNING MIND CONTROL

To begin with let us define the term mind control as we mean to use it. Mind control is the conscious ability to concentrate the mind toward a specific goal or on a specific muscle, with such determination and persistence that nothing will stop you or break your concentration. It is not a magical power to make you superman, or to move objects, change your life or personality. It is your will exercising itself on your conscious and subconscious mind to will it or make it perform and concentrate towards one specific object or idea.

The purposes of these exercises are to begin to exert the will on the mind and to begin to let the mind become more powerful in its ability to concentrate. When you are able to truly concentrate the power of the mind on the muscles of your body, the results can often be spectacular and serve not only as reinforcement to you of the power of the mind, but as convinces your muscles of the power the mind has over them. After all, your mind really controls the use of your muscles. The mind tells the muscles what to do and when to do it. The muscles do not control the mind and the mind is not limited by the muscles and their strength or lack of strength. The mind is potentially the most powerful weapon or force you have, and what you are doing now is training it to develop this power within it.

We have all heard the stories of the lady who picked the car off her son who was trapped under it, or of people who did other apparently superhuman things in time of great stress or excitement. They certainly did not become stronger in a flash and then lose it in the same flash. They only became more determined, more resolved, and concentrated on a job that had to be done immediately without hesitation. A matter of life and death, no other thoughts were in their minds except the action they were about to perform. After they did it they were just as amazed as your or I that they were able to do it. The mind has the potential to move mountains, whether by force, or by the invention of machines to blow the mountain up. Just as you give your mind exercises to make it smarter, you can give it exercises to make it stronger. For example, you give it math problems to learn to think abstractly; give it concentration feats (or Ki exercises) to teach it to grow more powerful.

In these exercises you are experiencing only positive reinforcement, you will not get hurt and you will not (if done according to instruction) ever experience a negative result. For example, when you are learning to have an unbendable wrist, you will never let your instructor bend your wrist, you stop him before he is able to. So the mind becomes programmed to expect to have only positive results and gradually becomes determined to have only Positive Results.

Unbendable Arm:

The Unbendable Arm. Just as a tree limb cannot be bent and water cannot be compressed, the arm is capable of not being bent when the mind directs it so. The first step is to concentrate the mind on the arm and to continue to reaffirm to the arm the fact. "This arm cannot be bent", next the arm should be placed on the shoulder of the partner and the partner should place both of his arms near the elbow joint and begin to try to bend the arm. The man trying not to have his arm bent must be careful not to roll the arm over and point the elbow up, for this assures that the arm cannot be bent but also that it can be broken. The student should project a mental image of himself walking forward and through the opponent. This should be practiced a little each day until such time as the arm cannot be bent by the partner. Both arms should be used. The ability to have unbendable arms can be very valuable in stiff arming an opponent in football and in throwing objects.

Steps in the "unbendable arm

1. Stand with the feet shoulder width apart and place your arm on the partners shoulder.

2. Pull him towards you so that you do not have to pull your arm out of socket, or extend it out, to reach him.

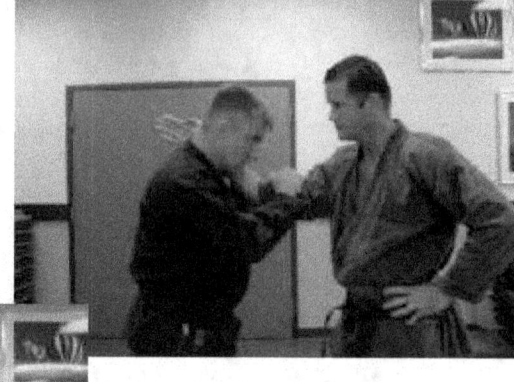

3. Affirm to yourself "this arm cannot be bent."

4. Let him begin to pull down on the arm, slowly, gradually increasing his pulling strength.

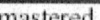

5. Slowly let your breath out, and let the arm bend slightly, with his pulling-down efforts.

6. Now assert your mind, your muscles and your breath and straighten the arm up and do not allow it to bend again.

7. Repeat with each arm daily until mastered.

8. When he is trying to bend your arm, if you feel it bending stop him and start over. Caution: do not roll the elbow up, this will break the arm. Do not let the partner jerk hard on the arm, let him pull slowly and steadily.

Results: Increase ability to concentrate; increased muscular control; increased confidence in yourself and your strength and ability; training of the mind to control the muscles; applicable to many sport situations (stiff arming in football, pushing weights, throwing objects in track and field, and the improved concentration that can be used in all sports).

Unbendable Wrist: Using an much mind control as possible and as little muscle as possible the student should attempt to hold his wrist straight and not let be bent backwards by the partner. One should exhale the breath during this trail and one should not let his wrist be bent while learning. In order to achieve this, when the student feels his wrist about to bend, he should tap his leg or say stop and then begin with his concentration again and another trial. This gives the student only positive reinforcement and will greatly improve his positive mental attitude. A projection of pushing the wrist straight up into the partners face should be concentrated upon also.

Steps in "unbendable wrist":

1. Stand with feet shoulder width and place your wrist in the partners hands.

2. Concentrate on the index finger and on the fact that your wrist "cannot be bent".

3. Slowly exhale your air, as the partner tries to bend your wrist backwards.

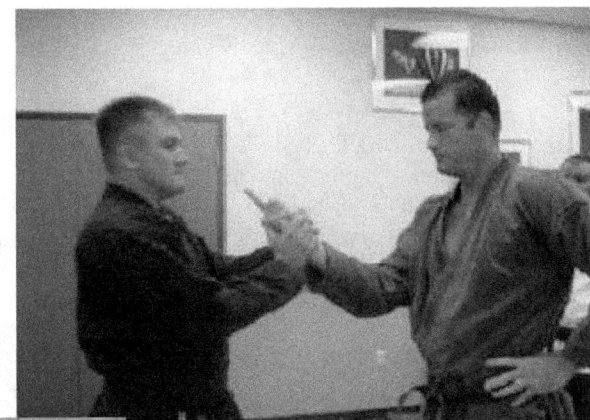

4. If you feel the wrist bending, stop the trial and begin a new one.

5. Imagine that you are pushing your wrist up into the sky, or into his face while he is trying to bend it.

11

6. Practice daily until mastered. (This should take a week to get to be able to do adequately, and 1 month to master.)

Cautions: Do not let the partner bend the wrist on the trials. This can hurt the wrist and give negative reinforcement.

Results: increased ability to concentrate; increased muscular control; increased confidence in your self; training of the mind to control the muscles.

Inseparable Arms:

Inseparable Arms. This is a simple matter of leverage, but serves to reinforce a positive mental attitude in the student. With the arms interlocked by the fingers and held at shoulder height, let two partners grab the student on the bicep area, not the forearm, and try to pull the arms apart. They should pull and not jerk and will find that they cannot pull them apart, even if as many as four men try to. Note: if a football is carried like this, it is impossible to be fumbled.

This exercise is primarily to show how people have been conditioned to misbelieve many things about the body. When the arms are placed in this position, they are actually already apart.

Note that the shoulders and elbows are

fully extended to the sides. The only thing that is together is the fingers and the partners are not trying to pull the fingers apart but the arms, which are already apart. So unless they jerk or pull from the front, they cannot pull the arms apart.

However this technique does have practical applications. If you wrap your arms around someone you wish to tackle in football, they will not be able to make you let your arms go. You may not tackle them, but at least they will drag you over the goal line and you won't look as bad as if you had let them go.

Arm on Head:

Arm on Head. Again the purpose of this exercise is to reinforce a positive mental attitude in the student, and can serve as a maneuver in sports (such as in basketball

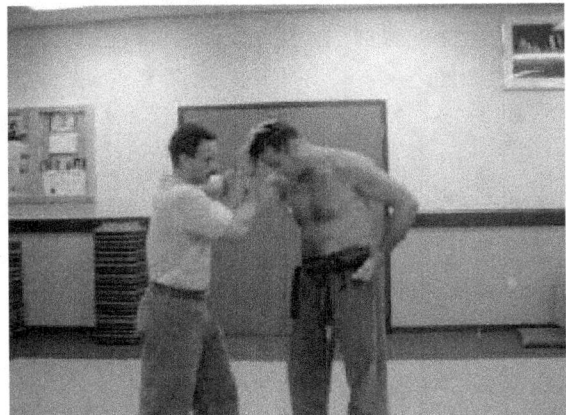

when the ball is grabbed from the backboard near the head). One will find that no matter how strong or powerful the partner, the arm cannot be separated from the top of the head, for it is quite easy to follow a downward pull and impossible for him to pull it off upwards.

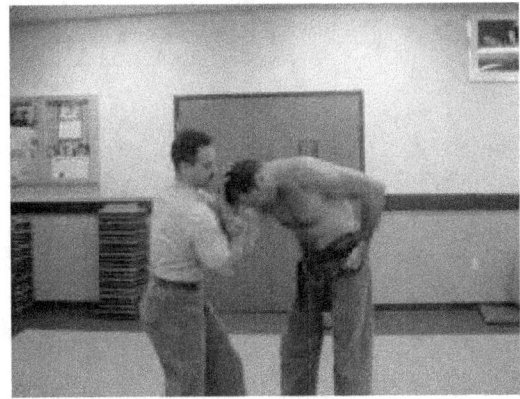

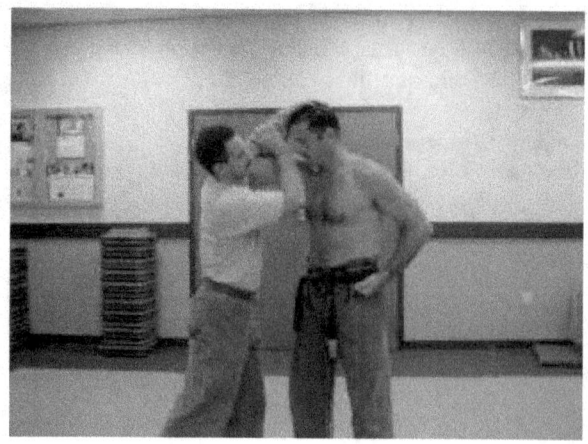

This ends the section on beginning mind control The student should practice these techniques until he has mastered them and has begun to exhibit some sort of conscious control over his mind without losing or breaking his concentration, or shown an ability to concentrate on one idea or one thought until he can do it perfectly.

TAKING A PUNCH IN THE STOMACH

You are now ready to begin to practice and apply your concept of KI by learning to take a punch in the stomach. We have already begun to practice all the three aspects that are necessary to develop our KI. We are doing sit ups, legs up and muscle conditioning exercises to strengthen the muscles and learn to control them. We are doing breathing exercises that enable us to concentrate on our breath and to as much as possible move it from various areas of our body that may be hit. We have practiced beginning mind control to learn to focus and concentrate the mind on one specific point, or to one area of the body. Now we will use all three at once and begin to see how easy it is to let someone hit us in the stomach without receiving an injury or even a bruise.

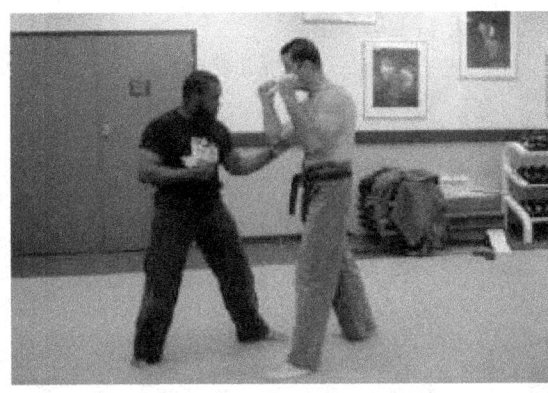

Taking   A   Punch in   the
Stomach:

1. Stand with the feet shoulder width apart and begin to concentrate the mind on the fact "I am going to get hit in the stomach". Keep affirming this fact over and over, at the same time asserting to yourself "I am not going to get hurt, I cannot be hurt by a hit in the stomach." Your mind is very strong and when concentrated it can achieve fantastic power. If it believes firmly that you are first of all; going to get hit in the stomach, it will prepare all the muscles of the body for the blow and will begin to concentrate the breath from the exercises you have been doing to control the breath. Next, when the mind tells your body "I am not going to get hurt" your body has no choice but to react as if it were not going to get hurt. Your muscles cannot think, your breath cannot think. They do not know if the person punching you can hurt you or not. Your mind must make that decision and you are conditioning your mind now by affirming to yourself the positive fact that you are not going to get hurt. Your mind will coordinate the muscles and the breath and prepare the body for the blow and the combination of the three factors will assure that you do not receive an injury. Note: you will never get hurt when practicing because first of all you will never be experiencing negative reinforcement, because you will be using a partner who will only punch you in the stomach the first time with his finger tips and will not hit you any harder till you are sure you can take a harder punch. Each time you train your confidence will be built up and each time your KI will become stronger because of your practicing it, you will not be getting hurt because of the light punches you are Taking while you are learning and by the time you are ready to let someone hit you very hard,
your mind is ready, your breath is ready, and your muscles are ready.

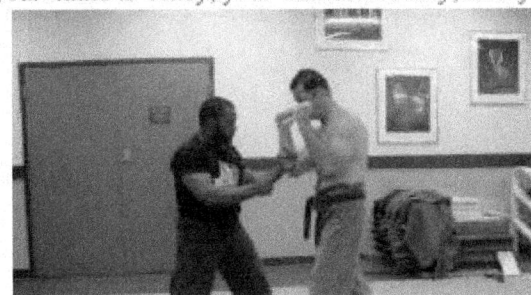

2.   Step forward   with either foot, and let half of the air out of the stomach area. Do not let all of the air out because the partner may wait until you

breathe in and then hit you. This can do damage. Let out half of
the air and continue to really concentrate the mind on the two important facts. "I
am going to get hit", and "I will not get hurt."

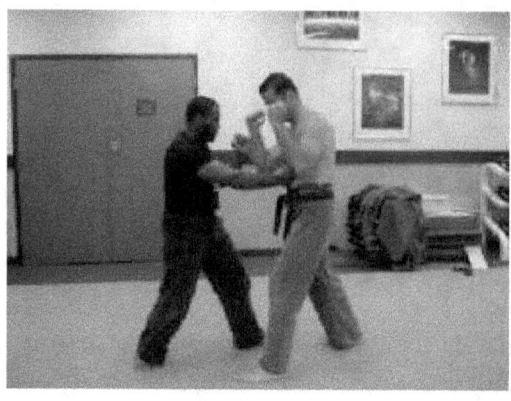

3. When you are firmly convinced in your mind that you are ready to take the punch and that you will not be hurt, nod your head and the partner will lightly hit you in the stomach. Keep your eyes open and as you see the punch coming, quickly begin to tighten all the stomach muscles and all the other muscles of the body. At the same time exhale all your air as forcefully as you can and make a noise when doing so. (The reason you make a noise is that you cannot let all your air out forcefully unless you are making a noise.) Some students are shy or reserved and do not want to make a loud noise. Let me assure you the louder the noise, the more power you are bringing into your stomach area - power of concentration, muscle control and breath.

4. When the punch hits your stomach, yell as loud as you can, tighten all the muscles and then keep the body and breath ready in case another punch is to follow. (Sometimes in a game you will get hit twice.) After you are certain no more punches are following, step back and smile, reconfirming to yourself that you were not hurt and you won't ever be hurt by these exercises. (This is to practice your positive conditioning.) Do not let the partner hit you several times in the beginning, unless you concentrate completely the mind each time as you did to take the first punch.

5. Each time you practice, you should increase the power of the punches that the partner is using and in a very short time you will be able to let him hit you as hard as he can without receiving any injury or bruise.

Review of Steps

First concentrate the mind on two facts:

"I am going to get hit in the stomach" and "I am not going to get hurt."

After you have accepted and believed these facts step forward and let out half of your breath. Continue your concentration and nod your head when you are ready for the partner to hit you.

At the instant of impact let out all your air as forcefully as you can, with a loud noise. Tighten every muscle of your body and believe that it can't hurt you.

Each time you can let him hit you harder but in the beginning it is not necessary or advisable to let him hit you with more than a tap, until you learn the proper technique for letting all your air out, tightening the muscles, and concentrating the mind.

Taking A Shot in The Ribs

Most of your life you have probably never had a coach, a friend or a teacher who ever told you what to do if you were going to get hit in the ribs. You may have been told to cover up, block it, get out of the way, but no one ever told you what you could do to protect the ribs if it were inevitable that you were going to get hit in the ribs. It is actually a most easy form of KI and can be learned quickly and applied easily to most game situations.

Remember that when you are getting hit in the ribs you are doing something, even if it is only letting your ribs get broken. Most people do exactly the wrong thing when they feel a hit coming into the ribs. They try to get out of the way. This does two bad things. It stretches the rib cage open and lets a lot of air into the chest. We have already seen that air can burst like a balloon, and certainly if you expose your ribs and separate them by leaning away from the blow, you will get them cracked or broken by the hit.

What you should do is to rely upon the three factors of your KI. Let the large muscle groups of the abdominal and the lats cushion and absorb most of the blow, at the same time let the breath be forcefully exhaled to keep the rib cage contracted as fully as possible and use the mind to concentrate your power to the area to make your muscles and breath react properly. If you do these three things the blow will just bounce off and cause no damage or pain.

Procedure: (when practicing place the hand on top of the head because in most games when you get hit in the ribs your arms are up, or out.)

1. Pull the lats muscle out as far as possible by concentrating the muscles of the latisumus dorsi and making them larger or expanded.

2. Lean the body to the side being hit, try to touch the elbow to your side, this squeezes the ribs together and protects them.

3. Let the breath out forcefully, to help you squeeze the ribs together and to contract the muscles.

4. Lean slightly forward in the area of the blow. This pulls the lats out further to act as a cushion for the blow.

If you are being punched in the floating ribs, (the area located at the sides of the abdominal muscles), you must lean forward, crunch down on the stomach and rib cage and into the blow. The stomach muscles play an important part in this KI and to fully get them tightened, and the ribs tightened, you must let your breath out at the point of impact as well as concentrate your mind.

Important: it is vital that you overemphasize the downward crunching movement of the ribs and the crunch of the stomach muscles.

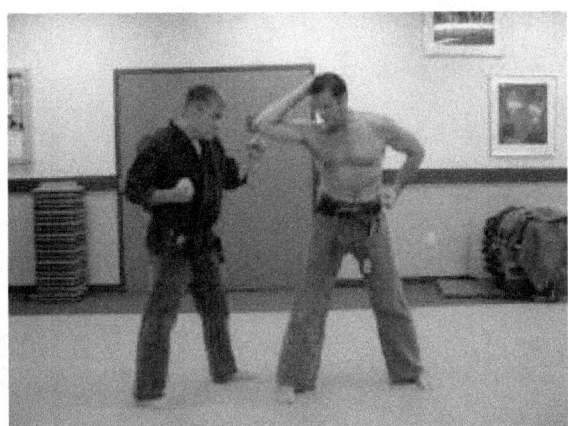

Taking a punch in the ribs:

    1. pull out the lats.

    2. lean into the punch.

    3. bend toward the punch.

    4. exhale the air at impact.

    5. concentrate the mind.

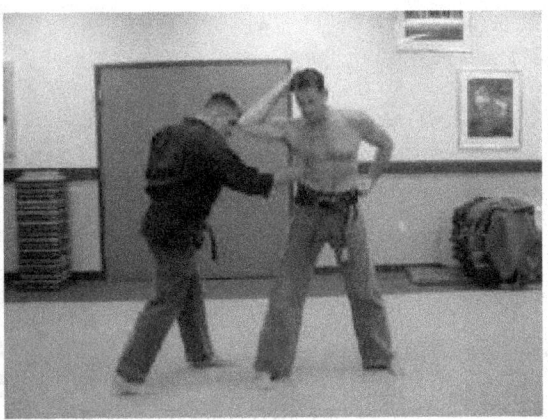

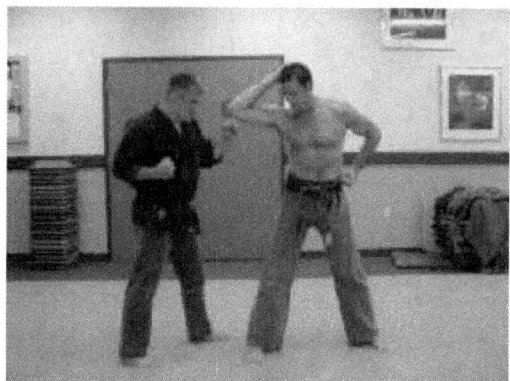

Taking an elbow in the ribs:

1. pull out the lat muscle.

2. lean toward the elbow.

3. bend toward the side.

4. exhale the air at the time of impact.

5. concentrate the mind.

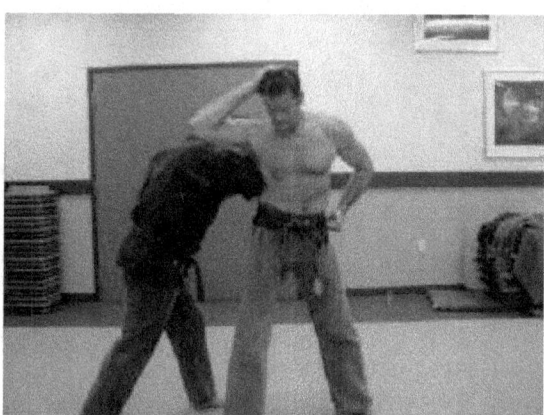

Strikes in The Neck

One of the most common and dangerous injuries that occurs in sports today is the neck injury. Many a weight lifting machine and numerous neck exercises have been invented and tried to strengthen the neck to help prevent the neck injury. But just making the neck stronger is like padding a glass jar and then repeatedly throwing it against the wall. Finally no matter how much padding someone will throw it just right and break the jar. So the same is true with the neck. The athlete often just tries to pad it more, or make it stronger and then keeps butting his head into other people and hitting his head against the wall. Finally one of the blows will be just right and the neck will get injured. It is a much better and safer idea to use your KI, to protect your neck and spine from injury. Remember, we are still relying heavily on the muscles to protect the neck, but now we are adding the protection of the breath and the concentration power of the mind.

Procedure for Taking a strike in the front of the throat or neck:

1. Tighten the neck muscles as tight as possible.

2. Jut the bottom jaw forward so that you have an under bite effect. At the same time pull back on the tongue and make the same muscle contraction you would use when you are swallowing.

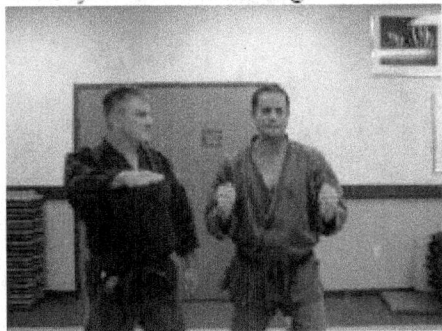

3. Lift the shoulders up and the traps muscles should be flexed. Tighten the fists to give strength to the trap and shoulder muscles.

4. Focus the mind on the fact that you are going to get struck in the neck and that you are not going to get hurt.

5. Breathe out slowly but extremely forcefully while you wait for the blow, at the instant of impact, really force your air through your neck (but do not make a sound or a noise other than the air escaping from your mouth).

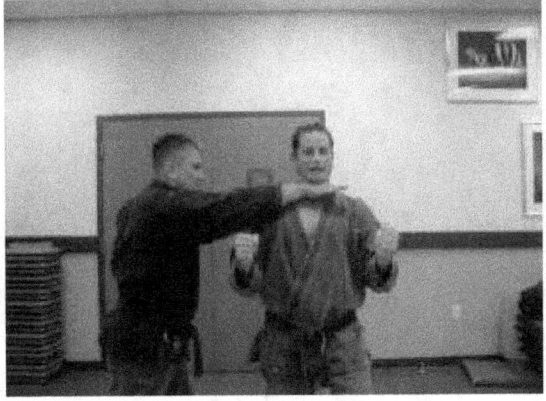

6. Keep the neck muscles and mind concentrated till you are sure no more blows are coming.

If you are doing this exercise correctly you can test to see if your neck is protecting itself by seeing if you have protected your adams apple area or larynx. To do this have your partner try to choke you. If you are doing the exercise correctly, your larynx should float back into the muscle area of your neck and be protected there. Do not bend your neck in such a fashion that your jaw rests on your chest because then you have not protected the neck, but exposed the jaw and teeth.

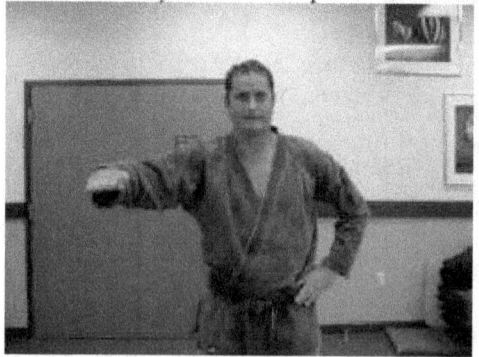 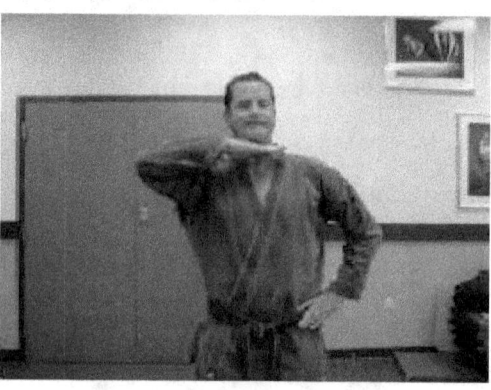

IMPORTANT...IF YOU CAN'T HIT YOURSELF IN THE THROAT AND NOT GET HURT, YOU CAN'T LET ANYONE ELSE HIT YOU IN THE THROAT.

DO NOT PRACTICE THROAT KI UNTIL YOU HAVE A THROUGH UNDERSTANDING OF MASTERY OF KI. YOU CAN GET KILLED.

If you are going to get struck in the **back of the neck**, you must do the following things in order to use your KI to protect your neck and spine.

1. Keep the back and spine as much as possible in a straight line. Do not be leaning forward or backwards.

2. Tighten all the muscles surrounding the neck for protection.

3. Exhale your breath forcefully to allow full muscle contraction and to aid your mind concentration.

4. Concentrate the mind very hard on the area being hit and firmly believe you will not be injured.

Notes: The neck can be protected by the use of KI but this is a very dangerous area to make a mistake in while practicing. I do not advise that you ever practice with full power blows to the front of the back of the neck, but rather practice with softer blows so that you can develop your technique and timing so that if you were hit there in the actual situation you could react fast enough and correctly.

Often you do not see the blows coming from behind to the back of the neck for the obvious reason that you do not have eyes in the back of your head. However you can be prepared for such blows as much as possible by getting into the habit of not relaxing the neck muscles and not leaning the neck forward or backwards.

The body position at the time of the impact from the strike in the neck. Note the jaw jutting forward, the neck being tightened and the concentration on the neck area.

A. 9 out of 10 times you do see the blow coming because it is illegal in most sports to hit the man from behind, and because you see the blow coming you will be able to react in time. Get in the habit of always being ready when on the field or playing. Don't let your guard down. Keep the muscles tense but not tight. Keep the breath under control. Do not get lazy and start breathing into stomach and keep the mind concentrated and prepared for a blow at any time. Remember the play is not over till you are in the huddle, the referee has the ball or the final gun has blown. I guess the best motto is to "Stay Prepared."

Q. How do I practice without getting hurt?

A. Practice in progressive steps using only positive reinforcement, start out with a tap, and only build up the power of the hits a very little at a time, as your technique progresses and your mind and body become stronger and more confident. So always use a partner that wants to help you learn, not one that wants to see you get hurt.

Q. How often should I practice my KI?

A. You should do your breathing exercises every day, your sit ups every day, your muscle training 3 times a week, your meditation and beginning mind control exercises every day for at least 3 months. By then you will have learned all the techniques well enough to take almost any blow without receiving an injury.

Then you may practice these exercises 3 times a week. Remember that your KI is as much technique as it is mind control and so you must practice your technique by letting people hit you. If you have not let anyone hit you for 4 weeks, your technique will not be as sharp, therefore your KI will not be as good. It is just like any sport, you must practice specific techniques quite often to stay in top condition.

Q. When should I not practice?

A. Do not try to do KI when you have been drinking. Alcohol deludes one into thinking he has more power than he really has; never when on drugs; or after eating - wait at least an hour; and do not try it just as you wake up, wait until you are fully awake and your mind is very clear. Also if you ever feel like you don't want to get hit, or just don't have any KI that day, then you are right and you should not practice your KI because you are not really doing KI for you have not got the absolute mind beliefs necessary to do it correctly.

Q. How do I do all these things in a game situation?

A. You already should have the muscle strength from your muscle training, and you can practice your breathing exercises before the game. Use the time you have in the huddle or before the ball is snapped or when you are on the sidelines to keep the mind concentration at a top level.

Procedure for Learning KI

Day One:

a. 50 sit ups, 50 leg ups, 20 side bends.

b. stomach breathing 2 minutes

c. isometric stomach breathing, 5 way

d. concentration for at least 30 seconds on "I am going to get hit in the stomach" and "I am not going to get hurt."

e. partner just jabs his fingers into solar plexus area (be sure to overact and really tighten the muscles, and scream at the instant of impact even though this is a soft blow.)

f. affirmation - affirm to yourself "that did not hurt, and I cannot get hurt by being punched in the stomach."

Day Two:

a. 60 sit ups, 60 leg ups, and 20 side bends.

b. stomach breathing 2 minutes.

c. isometric stomach - 5 way.

d. concentration for at least 30 seconds on the facts. "I am going to get hit." "I am not going to get hurt."

e. partner hits you in the stomach 1/4 of his full power. Be sure to overreact to the punch and greatly tighten the stomach muscles, forcefully exhale the air, and scream at the point of impact.

f. affirmation "that did not hurt, and I cannot get hurt by being punched in the stomach."

Day Three:

a. 70 sit ups, 70 leg ups, 20 side bends.

b. stomach breathing 2 minutes

c. isometric stomach - 5 way

d. concentration for at least 30 seconds (See above concentration thoughts)

e. partner hits you in the stomach 1/3 his power. Be sure to be over ready to this punch. In other words be ready for a punch twice that hard.

f. affirmation (see above affirmations)

Day Four:

a. 80 sit ups, 80 leg ups, 20 side bends.

b. stomach breathing 2 minutes

c. isometric stomach - 5 way

d. concentration for 30 seconds

d. partner hits you 1/2 power

e. affirmations

Day Five:

a. 90 sit ups, 90 leg ups, 20 side bends

b. stomach breathing 2 minutes

c. isometric stomach - 5 way

d. concentration for 30 seconds

e. partner hits you 2/3 power in stomach.

f. affirmations

Day Six:

a. 100 sit ups, 100 leg ups, 20 side bends.

b. stomach breathing 2 minutes

c. isometric stomach - 5 way

d. concentration for as long as you need to take a full power punch. Not more than a minute should be needed.

e. partner hits you as hard as he can in the stomach.

f. affirmations and congratulations by partner and coach.

Rest Sunday.

The second week continue to do 100 sit ups, 100 leg ups, and 20 side bends a day. 2 minutes of stomach breathing, 5 way isometric stomach, try to lessen the amount of time you need to concentrate, and begin to practice your Rib KI in the same gradual manner you did the stomach KI. By the end of the week you should be able to take a full power punch in the stomach and a fully power strike in the ribs.

Week 3. Continue to do 100 sit ups, 100 leg ups, 20 side bends, 2 minutes stomach breathing, 5 way isometric stomach, increase your concentration ability, take punches in stomach and ribs, and begin to practice techniques for neck KI (but do not practice Taking hard strikes in the neck EVER, just practice the technique.)

You should continue to practice your KI vigorously and religiously every day you can until you have developed the techniques so that you are able to let someone punch you either in the ribs, or the stomach without more than a split seconds notice, and until you can take several strikes in a row to different areas of your body. Your KI will get better every day, as your mind gets stronger and you breath and muscle control becomes sufficient so that you are absolutely assured of their immediate full cooperation when you practice your KI.

KI will work. KI does work. KI can be developed by you, or by anyone who is willing to do the training required and to believe in themselves. You must not neglect a single exercise. You must be able to do 100 sits ups, 100 leg ups, and 20 side bends. You should develop a regular muscle strengthening program. 2 minutes of stomach breathing every day for at least a month. Isometric stomach breathing 5-way, beginning mind control exercises and meditation techniques all must be mastered. Progressive-positive training with the proper partner and you will soon be a master of Hard KI.

REMOVAL OF PAIN & AVOIDANCE OF PAIN

To begin with we must understand what pain is and what the purpose of pain is. Pain is a defense mechanism used by the body to warn it that an injury is occurring, or has occurred, and to keep it alert to the injured to the injured area to avoid re-injuring it. Pain is not caused by the injury but is caused by the nerves reacting to the injury. The science of acupuncture and acupressure has developed techniques to stop the nerves from transmitting pain to the brain and thereby stop the brain from feeling the sensation of pain. Pain must therefore be interpreted by and felt in the brain. Even though it seems as though the injury is being felt in the area of the damage, what is in fact happening is the pain is being sent to the brain via the nerves, translated and interpreted in the brain and sent back to the affected area. A cycle is thus formed with the nerves and the brain. Not with the injury and the brain. It is not necessary to experience pain unless the pain is being experienced by the actual injury occurring. So we have developed drugs in America to stop the pain from being interpreted in the brain. The aspirin is the most popular, and all the way up to Heroin which is so strong that you can have surgery without any pain being experienced during the operation.

So you can also learn techniques for avoiding the sensation of pain or preventing and removing the pain syndrome. These techniques are not new and have been used by the Orientals for thousands of years and by many American athletes and individuals who perhaps may not have been aware exactly what they were doing.

When you were young you used a similar technique for the removal of pain. Remember when you would fall down and hurt your knee. You would grab your knee and take a deep breath, squeeze your muscles, then limp home and your mother would kiss it and make it well. Usually you really did feel better and most of the pain was gone. What was happening was the use of three techniques for the removal or avoidance of pain that we will use. You were using breath control, muscle control and mind control. You used your breath to draw your body's healing powers to the area and to stop the nerve movement. You used your muscle to tighten the area and draw extra blood into it and relieve some of the pain. You used your mother's kiss as a mental affirmation that you no longer hurt.

Let us see some techniques that can be applied to slight injuries that often occur in sports. Note: you can use these techniques for major injuries such as a broken bone or wounds, but we are concerned with injuries that you have that are minor and that if you were not affected by the pain you could continue to play and perform at top level.

Joint Injuries: Slight sprains and jams.

1. Take a deep breath and tighten the muscles that have been hurt. Now hold your breath while directing your mind to send your breath to the area that is hurt. (Of course you can't send air to the area, only suggest to your mind that you are sending your breath with its healing properties to the injured area.)

2. Make circles, pointing away from the heart, around the affected area, not on the affected area. Rub around it about 5-10 times then mentally take the pain into your finger tips and throw it away with a flick of your fingers - away from the body. (You can't actually throw away the pain, but you can give your mind and your body the autosuggestion that you are throwing away the pain.)

3. Forget that you are injured and pay no more attention to any pain that may still be coming to the brain. Begin to concentrate very hard on the task or game at hand. Do not let the mind wander to the sensation of pain. Forget it, do not notice it. (Just like a man that works in a noisy factory learns not to notice the noise after he has been there a while.) Don't worry that you may re-injure the area or that if you do your mind control may not let you notice the pain, just like the man in the factory who does not notice the noise, he immediately notices something going wrong, or a strange sound, so you will too notice any further injury.

Jammed thumb or sprained finger:

a. rub around the area

b. take a deep breath

c. tighten the muscles for a few seconds

d. throw away the pain

e. forget the pain

Slightly sprained ankle

a. rub around the ankle

b. take a deep breath

c. tighten the muscles for a few seconds

d. throw away the pain

e. forget the pain

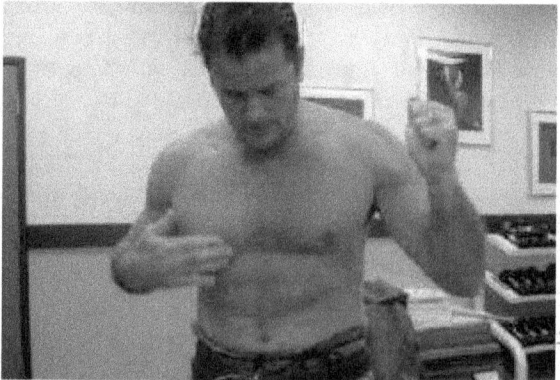

Throwing away the pain and forgetting the pain or

techniques that take practice and that take concentration and belief in ones mind control. But more importantly it takes the desire of the athlete not to let an injury affect his performance or stop his performance. A great athlete is usually playing with some kind of pain and to get to be the best

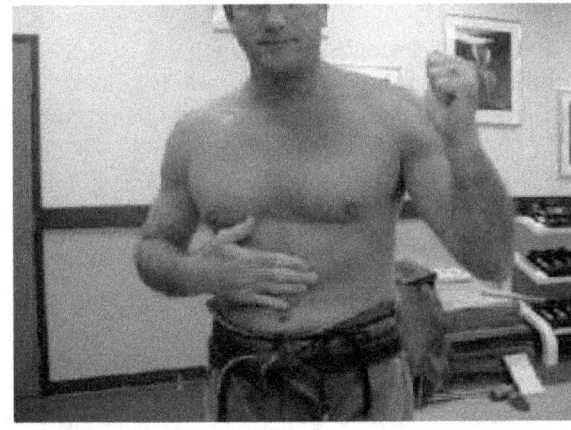

Throwing away the pain in the ribs you have to undergo much pain and trial with pain to perfect your game and technique. Believe you can stop the pain, desire to stop the pain and to go on playing and you will certainly develop this technique.

Throwing away and stopping pain in the ribs or stomach area.

RELAXATION

The ability to relax cannot be overemphasized and can be defined for our use to mean the ability to leave the game out of your body, but keep it in your mind. Too many coaches and players lose points, games and get ulcers because they cannot control their tempers or attitudes during the game situation. They have let their reactions be determined by the actions of other people, referees, or players. Therefore, they find themselves like puppets on a string, ranting and raving, or awkward and clumsy because they have destroyed the delicate relationship between the body and the mind. They have let their emotions take a disproportionate part in their actions and because of that they have lost their style, poise and grace. We have all seen far too many cases of this and know it's true. (For example: the coach in the ball game who runs up and down the side lines, kicking the ground and the players and screaming and shouting at the referee, the player who can't make a shot because he is so nervous and anxiety ridden, the player who jumps off sides several times or who starts fights for the slightest provocation.) The problem with these people is that they have lost control of their body by letting their mind become confused and disoriented. Your mind cannot think of two things at once and do a good job on either one. You must have a calm mind if you want to make the shot, or to think the play out. Your mind tells and directs your muscles to perform as they have been conditioned but if your mind is racing between being upset and making the shot, being angry and being relaxed then the muscles get contradictory information to them and subsequently do not perform as programmed but become dis-coordinated. The brain becomes confused by the huge influx of emotional stimulus and can't reason intelligently, perform adequately and begins to send out all kinds of emergency signals to the body. You see, your mind cannot distinguish between a vividly imagined event and an actual occurrence. So when you begin to think angry, your brain interprets danger and sends out the appropriate body responses. Your adrenaline starts to be released, thereby causing the blood pressure to go up, the heart beats faster, the stomach stops digesting and begins secreting acid, the eyes dilate and the muscles become jerky and tensed. So your body is prepared for attack or defense and when none comes the damage is irreversible. No one is easier to handle than a drunk, or a man that has gone crazy and so angry that he is like a wild man, he obviously can't perform his primary function in the game and so your defense or offensive gets the advantage of having one more player on their side functioning at peak condition and one less on your side not only functioning poorly but probably causing others to perform badly. Ulcers and lost games, fights and lost friends are just some of the results of the inability to relax.

Any great athletic performance seems effortless because the athlete has practiced and practiced until he has programmed his body for the appropriate response. He has learned to keep his mind calm and to relax while performing, thereby conserving his energy and assuring a longer and better performance. He is like a work of art, graceful and beautiful to look at, because he has achieved harmony between his body and mind. A great coach is the same thing. He has learned to teach and train his team with patience, kindness and understanding. He has confidence in his team and his coaching staff. He knows that they will do the best that they can, and that the game is not the time to change previously conditioned responses or to try to do a coaching job that should have been done in practice sessions. So he remains calm and relaxed on the sidelines and usually winds up winning. Of course there are coaches who become involved to a great extent and are also winners, but they don't last as long and generally pay for their involvement with ulcers and loss of friends and support. No one likes you when you are upset especially your own body. So let's practice a form of relaxation that takes only 3 minutes and can be as beneficial as 1 hour of sleep.

Relaxation Technique: lie on the floor with the feet together and the palms face down on the sides of the body. Look straight up and do not move the eyes. This is important. Now take a deep breath, hold it for a second and tighten the feet. Now relax and exhale. As you do, say mentally to yourself, "relax, my feet are relaxed." Now take a deep breath and tighten the calves. old the tension a second. As you release the breath say gently to yourself "my calves are relaxed." Take another deep breath and tighten the thighs. Hold it for a second. As you release the breath, relax the thighs.

Your legs are now completely relaxed. You no longer wish to move your legs. You could move your legs, but you no longer wish to move them. Take a deep breath into your stomach, hold it. As the air leaves your stomach, relax your stomach. Now breathe deeply into your lungs. As the air leaves your lungs, relax your chest and let your breath become very subtle and soft. Now breathe and tighten the arms and hands. Hold the tension a second. Then relax. As the breath leaves your arms become very relaxed. Your entire body is now very relaxed and you feel as if you are floating on a cloud, very calm and very relaxed. Take a breath and tighten your neck and shoulders. Hold it and as you let your breath out relax your neck area. Now take a breath and make a large frown, an ugly face. Now relax and breathe out, and relax your face, more and more till your jaw almost drops open. Your entire body is now completely relaxed and you feel extremely calm and relaxed. The only thing left to relax are your eyes. Gently close your eyes. You should immediately start dreaming now.

Just let your mind roam and relax, dream of soft and nice things. Imagine you are floating on a raft in a calm lake, or sailing on a cloud. Relax and feel the air flow through your body, relax and dream. Relax and dream. Let the mind float from one thought to the next, paying no special attention to any thought. Just watch them come and go in the mind like you see cars come and go on the highway. Relax and think of beautiful things. Think of nature, music, art, of love. Relax and feel yourself floating.

Now when one wishes to come out of this relaxed atmosphere, one should not just jump up. Gently open the eyes and take a deep breath and move the fingertips and the toes, breathe again and move the arms and the legs, breathe again and bend the arms and legs, and move the hips. Now take the arms and rub the back of the neck and calmly sit up and relax in a meditative posture for a few more seconds. You will feel very relaxed and quite calm and refreshed. This is truly a valuable way of letting an athlete relax and should be used by all serious students.

Three minutes of this relaxation is better for the body than 1 hour of sleep because it calms the nerves, refreshes the spirit, and soothes the mind. It is fast and simple to do and can be used after a workout or running (three minutes of sitting on the side of the track with the head between the legs trying to regain the breath after running does very little to relax you, while three minutes of this exercise does wonders.)

You can do this exercise lying down and it is very helpful to those who have trouble going to sleep. You can also do this standing up or sitting down during the game on the sidelines. As a coach, just take a few deep

breaths and tighten the muscles just as if you were lying down. In a few breaths you will begin to become calm and feel more relaxed. Just close your eyes for a few seconds and suggest to yourself a few pleasant thoughts. Your mind should become calm and relaxed and subsequently your performance as a coach and player will be at its strongest point.

The mind cannot be relaxed and calm when the body is breathing fast and furiously. So the necessity of regaining control over your breath as soon as possible after exertion is very important. Often when we run, we begin to experience anoxia and we get too much blood pumping too much oxygen and lose the delicate balance between good and bad air in our bodies. So we must use our mind to control our breathing and slow our breathing to allow the oxygen, carbon dioxide stages to be equalized.

Deep Breathing, or Circular Breathing:

To be used when you find yourself breathing too fast after exercise or after you exert yourself to assure that your muscles are getting an adequate supply of air.

Stand with the feet shoulder width apart and touch the hands together in front of the body. Begin the breath very slowly and easily as the arms are lifted up in a clockwise circle around the head and down the sides of the body, continuing to breathe in air the entire circle. Do this three times and one will feel much more refreshed and have a much more adequate air supply to necessary muscles. As you practice doing this exercise, you will learn to control your breathing and be able to get more benefit from the circular breathing. It is the fastest and easiest way to regain the proper breathing control after running or strong physical exertion.

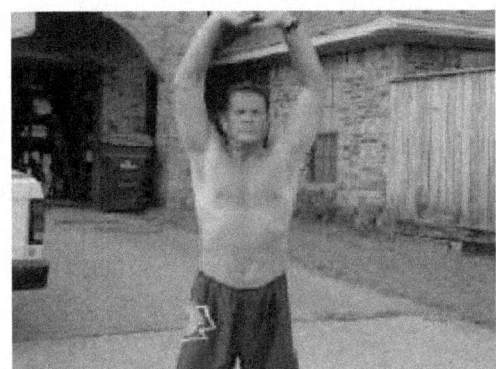

Raise the arms above the head and as you pull the arms down around your body, breathe in very deeply.

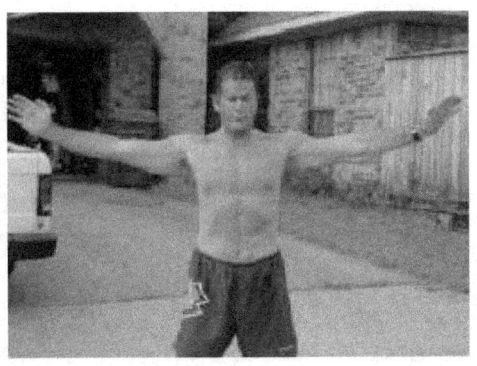

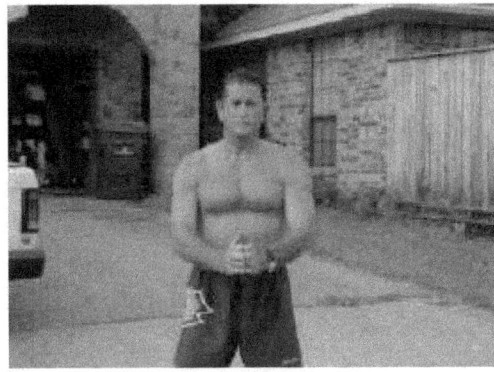

As you continue your circle breath out and you bring your arms back up to the top.

35

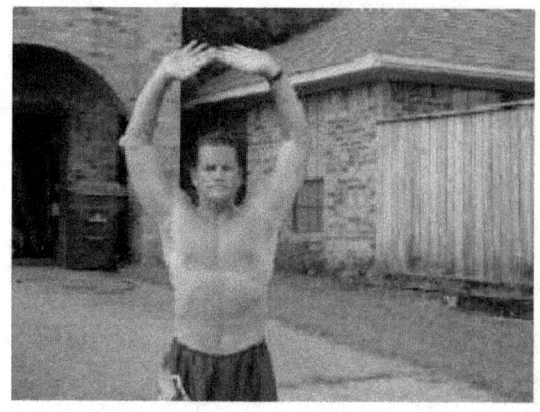

BREATHING EXERCISES

The breath plays a most important part in the relaxing of the body and often it is the breath that is the determiner of the body's responses, not the body that is determining the breath's reaction. In other words you are not breathing fast because you have been running, you are able to run because you are able to breathe quickly and supply the additional oxygen requirements to the body. You could not run at all if you could not breathe at all. In fact, you could not do anything at all if you could not breathe well. You would be asthmatic and unable to perform any vigorous exercise or to exert too much.

Your breath is the most important thing in your body. It is the only thing that you can not consciously deprive yourself of. You can poke your eyes out, kill yourself for love, bust your ear drums listening to loud music, deprive yourself of food, but you cannot hold your breath till you suffocate and you cannot let someone else suffocate you. Your body will not just relax and let itself be deprived of air. You will do anything to anyone when the need for air becomes dire for your survival.

The breath plays a very important part in relaxation because it plays a large part in the control of our body's reactions to certain events. For example, we have already noted that we could not run if we were not able to breathe fast and deep enough to supply the additional oxygen requirement needed by the body. When we are angry our breath becomes short and fast like when we are running. But when we are sleeping, our breath becomes slow and deep and relaxed and so is our mind. We cannot be breathing slow and deep and relaxed if we are angry. Just as we cannot be breathing slow and easy when we are upset. We breathe calm and our mind responds calmly, our muscles respond calmly. Your breath stills the mind and calms the nerves. So exercises have been developed centuries ago by people who understood the importance of the breath as a factor in self understanding and mind and body control. We will practice or study by practice, three of these methods.

Counting the Breaths: Sit in a meditative posture (see Chapter 10) and take a few deep breaths to calm the mind. Now begin to concentrate only on the breath as it comes in and as it leave the body. Try to clear the mind of all outside thoughts and concentrate only on the incoming and outgoing breaths. When you begin to breathe in, think only of the number One or only of this being your first breath. Let no other thoughts enter your mind but the number One. Continue to concentrate on this number all the way through the breath and as you begin to breathe out, continue to think and concentrate only on the number One. Now as you begin your next breath think and concentrate only on the number Two. Clear the mind of all other thoughts and think only of the number Two as you breathe in and as your breathe out. Continue to do this slow breathing and concentration up to the number Ten striving to keep the mind calm, not tense, and concentrating only on the numbers.

In a very few seconds you will see the extreme difficulty of clearing the mind and in only concentrating on the numbers. Thoughts will begin to float up and your mind will notice them and you will begin to feel and think about these thoughts and so become distracted from your primary purpose of thinking and seeing only the numbers. But do not become discouraged. This is an exercise and technique that can take literally years of practice to do perfectly. The mind is always full of extra thoughts and you must practice trying to calm it just as you would practice trying to learn a new skill, over and over again with patience and a calm and resolved manner. You cannot still the mind by being angry at it for thinking other thoughts, or calm the mind by tightening the muscles. Just relax and try to concentrate the mind only on the breath. Gradually you will be able to think only of the numbers.

Counting The Breath 2. If you are having great difficulty in visualizing the numbers then perhaps the visualization of colors will be easier for you. when you breathe in, think only of the color red, through the entire breath, and then of the color blue, then green, then orange, then black, then white, then yellow, then brown, then purple, and finally pink, (or you can use any color you wish). This may be easier for you and provides a more pleasing visual stimulus for the mind.

You should perform this counting exercise every day for at least a few weeks until you have begun to gain some mastery over your mind and some control of your mind. Practice should only take a few minutes, up to five, and so should not be troublesome to you for finding the time to practice. After you have begun to get good in this you may want to do it more often for the relaxing effects it has on the mind and body. You may do it as often or as little as you wish. You can do it on the sidelines when you find yourself getting upset (remember how your mother told you to count to ten if you were angry). The same effect is achieved now but you are adding the effect of the slow and easy breathing to calm the nerves and soothe the mind.

Controlling The Breath: this exercise trains one in the voluntary control of the breath by the conscious will of the mind. You will not be allowing the body to breathe normally but will be trying to force it to breathe as the mind wishes.

Sit in the meditative posture and close the eyes. Take a few deep breaths to calm the mind and now slowly begin to breathe in for the count of 10, count each number silently to yourself. Now hold your breath without pressing down or lifting your shoulders up for the count of 10. Now begin to breathe out for the count of 10, trying to make the out-breathing slow and controlled and not breathe out all the air at the beginning of the out-breath. Immediately after you have breathed out for 10, begin to breathe in again for the count of 10. Hold it for 10 and out for 10. Do this exercise 10 times. You will find that you may start to sweat and that you really have to use a lot of muscles and mind control to stop your body from breathing in too quickly or out too fast. This is an excellent form of breathing control and the benefits are numerous. It teaches the mind great strength and begins to reconfirm to the muscles the power of the mind over them. It produces a body heat, and so can be used if you are cold; and it strengthens the breath control by the actual controlling g of the breathing movement. You can consider yourself exceptional if you can breathe in for 30 seconds, hold it for 30 seconds and breathe out for 30 seconds - 10 times. This shows a true mastery of the breath and a great deal of muscle and mind control. Do this exercise daily for a few weeks until you have been able to do all ten breaths in the correct count. Thereafter you may do it as often as you wish for the benefits to the muscles, the body and the mind.

Following The Breath: the purpose of this exercise is to transcend the mind and to concentrate only on the breath as it fills the body and the lungs and to follow it as it comes and goes in and out. This is a very soothing and relaxing form of breathing and the benefits are long lasting and comforting.

Sit in the meditative posture, close the eyes and take a few deep breaths to calm the mind and relax the nerves. Now as you begin to breathe in, try to let all other thoughts leave the mind except following the breath as it goes through your nostrils, down your throat and fills your lungs, then is dispersed to the various parts of your body. Follow it as it returns up your throat and out your nostrils and into the air. Try to imagine a golden string being attached to your lungs that comes out of you as you breathe the air out and comes back into the lungs as you breathe in. Let your mind remain calm and follow the breath softly and easily. Soon you will begin to feel the body become filled with air and begin to feel very calm and relaxed, very soothed and light. The breath will fill your mind and your body and you will begin to feel as light as your breath itself. Do this exercise as long as you feel light and are able to concentrate on following the breaths. It is very soothing and relaxing. Perform this exercise any time you are upset or any time you wish to feel truly relax

THE TIGER EYE

The "Tiger Eye" is a term that we will use to mean peripheral vision, or the ability to see everything that is surrounding you without the necessity of moving the eyes or the head. This technique is very valuable in most sports and causes an increase in awareness and subsequently performance. If you can see everything that surrounds you, the chances of your throwing an interception, or missing a tackle or shot are greatly reduced.

The Meditative Position: there are as many different positions for meditation (or concentration on a specific thought towards a specified goal) as there are forms of meditation. All have their benefits but some of them are difficult to get into position to do. So we will use a simple but effective position, called in Yoga the half lotus position.

Sit on the floor with the legs crossed in front of the body. Place the right leg in first and cross the left leg in front of that. Strive to keep the knees as near the ground as possible and the back, spine and neck in a straight line. Rock back and forth and gently to the sides to assure you are sitting up straight. Place the arms on the tops of the knees with the palms up. This helps to stabilize and balance the back. You may feel uncomfortable in this position. That is because you are not flexible enough. To improve flexibility do the stretches found in the front of the book, but if you are not flexible because you have not been doing the stretches long enough you may modify the position so that you are grabbing the knees or even putting the legs straight out. You may even sit in a straight backed chair while you are learning your flexibility.

The half lotus position. Note the straight back, the arms on the knees, the left leg in front of the right, and the steady and calm eyes.

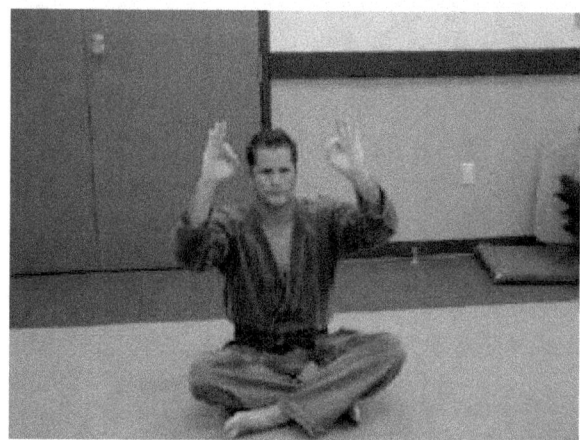

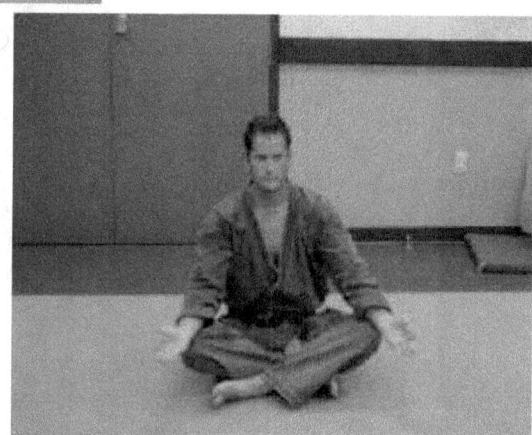

One should sit in the half lotus position while practicing the Tiger Eye and the gaze should be straight ahead with the eyes not moving to fix a point for the gaze.

The hands should be held above the head to start with, the fingers forming a triangle, and then slowly brought down to in front of the eyes. There the eyes should be fixed in their gaze upon one area and no longer move. The hands should then be placed on the knees, palms up with the thumb and forefinger inter joined. Now the Tiger Eye should be practiced.

After one has assumed the meditative posture one should fix the gaze of his eyes directly ahead and on one point. Let us assume you are looking at a football field during a game and you are standing in the middle of the field facing the goal line. Now without moving your eyes you can see the following things. You can see the goal posts and the end zone. You can see the stripes on the field and the grass, and the colors of the grass. You can see the sidelines, and the benches full of other players on the sidelines. You can see the players on the playing field, all of the players, and you can see the sky. You can see the lights around the stadium and the fans in the seats around the stadium. You can see the players directly beside you and across from you. In other words, you can see everything - in front of you, on the side of you, above you, and below your feet.

Now listen, you can hear the crowd. You can hear the sports announcer. You can hear the coach and players yelling on the sidelines. You can hear the quarterback and the players on the field talking, and even walking or hitting each other on the plays. You can see everything and you can hear everything going on around you. This is total awareness, total visual and sensory awareness. You cannot be surprised by a clip, or scared by a yell of another player. You are aware, just like the tiger is aware in the jungle. Yet you are relaxed and ready to move in any direction at any time, just like the tiger in the jungle.

You will find upon investigation that when the eyes are looking straight ahead and not focusing too sharply on one particular object that all the field of vision can be seen. But if you move your eyes side to side very fast or move your head quickly, then everything becomes blurred and you can actually not see things clearly. Just like a good hunter only looks at the trees and notices the slightest movement, not at the individual limbs and sees only that limb. Just imagine that the field is like a small painting. You can see all of the painting clearly but not if you are moving your head from side to side or your eyes quickly from side to side. So try to get in the habit of moving the whole body when you move the eyes. That way you are always keeping the vision clear and the body in such a position to react accordingly and effectively. (for example, if you look out the corner of your eye, you can see. But if someone was going to hit you and you could just see him in the corner of your eye, your body would not be in a very strong position for defending yourself. It is better to turn the whole body to look.) before, and you will thus be practicing your peripheral vision and soothing the nerves and calming the mind. The more you become aware of the things around you, the more you begin to appreciate them and their beauty.

The "Tiger Eye" is most useful for foul shooting, quarterbacks, safeties, and linebackers and for coaching (for all good coaches are able to look at the play and see the whole play unfolding at once, not just one player at a time. So a spotter who uses this technique will be a more effective spotter because he will be able to see the whole field and whole play at once.)

The "Tiger Eye" also involves listening for when you are relaxed and noticing all the sights around you, you are also noticing all the sounds around you. A good player is not drawn off sides by the change in the quarterback's cadence or inflection, and a good player does not lose concentration when the crowd boos him or is screaming at him or the team. He is just concentrating on the shot, or the game. He hears the noise but is not distracted by it.

You can practice the Tiger Eye while walking around school or at home. Just look straight ahead when you walk and do not move the eyes. You will see all the people coming and going around you and any movement to the right and left. You will feel calm and hear things you have not noticed

To begin with we must understand what pain is and what the purpose of pain is. Pain is a defense mechanism used by the body to warn it that an injury is occurring, or has occurred, and to keep it alert to the injured to the injured area to avoid re-injuring it. Pain is not caused by the injury but is caused by the nerves reacting to the injury. The science of acupuncture and acupressure has developed techniques to stop the nerves from transmitting pain to the brain and thereby stop the brain from feeling the sensation of pain. Pain must therefore be interpreted by and felt in the brain. Even though it seems as though the injury is being felt in the area of the damage, what is in fact happening is the pain is being sent to the brain via the nerves, translated and interpreted in the brain and sent back to the affected area. A cycle is thus formed with the nerves and the brain. Not with the injury and the brain. It is not necessary to experience pain unless the pain is being experienced by the actual injury occurring. So we have developed drugs in America to stop the pain from being interpreted in the brain. The aspirin is the most popular, and all the way up to Heroin which is so strong that you can have surgery without any pain being experienced during the operation.

So you can also learn techniques for avoiding the sensation of pain or preventing and removing the pain syndrome. These techniques are not new and have been used by the Orientals for thousands of years and by many American athletes and individuals who perhaps may not have been aware exactly what they were doing.

When you were young you used a similar technique for the removal of pain. Remember when you would fall down and hurt your knee. You would grab your knee and take a deep breath, squeeze your muscles, then limp home and your mother would kiss it and make it well. Usually you really did feel better and most of the pain was gone. What was happening was the use of three techniques for the removal or avoidance of pain that we will use. You were using breath control, muscle control and mind control. You used your breath to draw your body's healing powers to the area and to stop the nerve movement. You used your muscle to tighten the area and draw extra blood into it and relieve some of the pain. You used your mother's kiss as a mental affirmation that you no longer hurt.

Let us see some techniques that can be applied to slight injuries that often occur in sports. Note: you can use these techniques for major injuries such as a broken bone or wounds, but we are concerned with injuries that you have that are minor and that if you were not affected by the pain you could continue to play and perform at top level.

Joint Injuries: Slight sprains and jams.

1. Take a deep breath and tighten the muscles that have been hurt. Now hold your breath while directing your mind to send your breath to the area that is hurt. (Of course you can't send air to the area, only suggest to your mind that you are sending your breath with its healing properties to the injured area.)

2. Make circles, pointing away from the heart, around the affected area, not on the affected area. Rub around it about 5-10 times then mentally take the pain into your finger tips and throw it away with a flick of your fingers - away from the body. (You can't actually throw away the pain, but you can give your mind and your body the autosuggestion that you are throwing away the pain.)

3. Forget that you are injured and pay no more attention to any pain that may still be coming to the brain. Begin to concentrate very hard on the task or game at hand. Do not let the mind wander to the sensation of pain. Forget it, do not notice it. (Just like a man that works in a noisy factory learns not to notice the noise after he has been there a while.) Don't worry that you may re-injure the area or that if you do your mind control may not let you notice the pain, just like the man in the factory who does not notice the noise, he immediately notices something going wrong, or a strange sound, so you will too notice any further injury.

Jammed thumb or sprained finger:

a. rub around the area

b. take a deep breath

c. tighten the muscles for a few seconds

d. throw away the pain

e. forget the pain

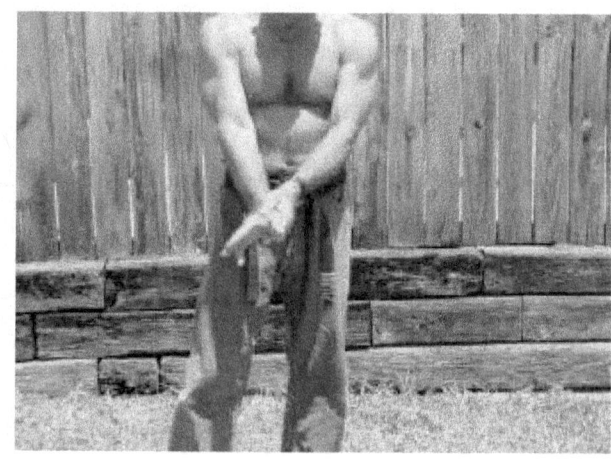

Slightly sprained ankle

a. rub around the ankle

b. take a deep breath

c. tighten the muscles for a few seconds

d. throw away the pain

e. forget the pain

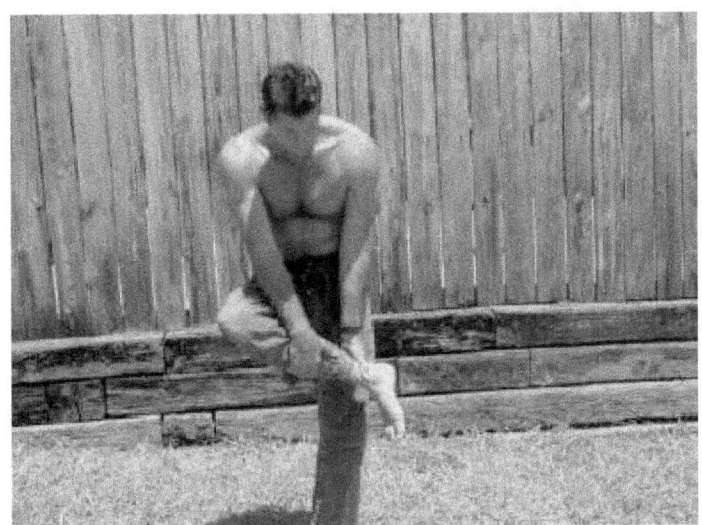

Throwing away the pain and forgetting the pain or techniques that take practice and that take concentration and belief in ones mind control. But more importantly it takes the desire of the athlete not to let an injury affect his performance or stop his performance. A great athlete is usually playing with some kind of pain and to get to be the best

Throwing away the pain in the ribs you have to undergo much pain and trial with pain to perfect your game and technique. Believe you can stop the pain, desire to stop the pain and to go on playing and you will certainly develop this technique.

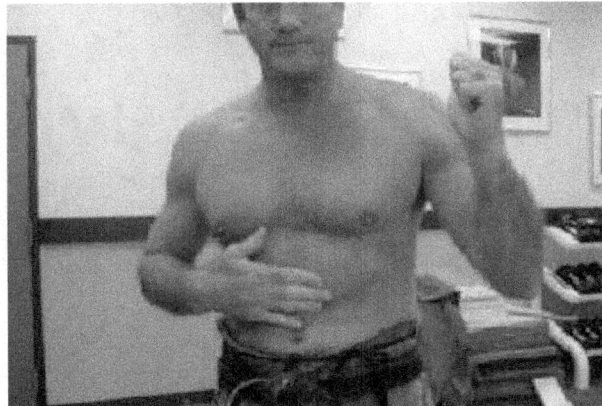

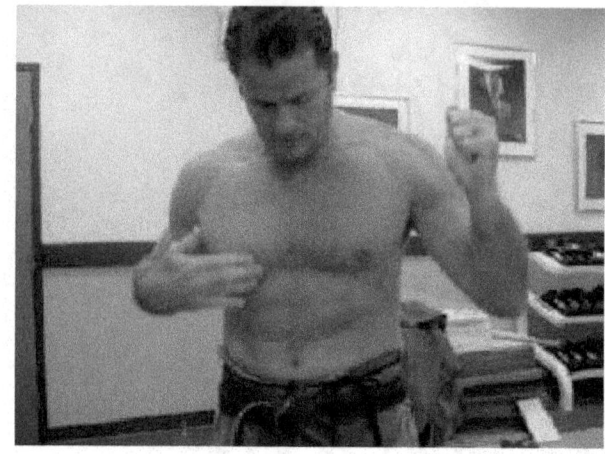

Throwing away and stopping pain in the ribs or stomach area.

Chapter 7

FALLING

Perhaps no other and more obvious aspect of injuries that can be prevented is being taught less or understood less by the coaches and players in America than the proper method to fall on the ground without being injured. I am not talking about rolling forward, which is what most people think falling is. I am referring to getting your feet knocked out from under you and going 4 feet in the air and landing on your shoulder or neck, or being tackled or knocked down sideways and breaking your wrist, or slipping on the snow or ice and falling on your butt and injuring your tail bone or neck. These are examples of falls that athletes are constantly being exposed to, and that they are usually not at all prepared to negotiate or execute without receiving injury. For too long players, coaches, and fans have expected that if a players feet are taken out from under him, or he is thrown into the air, he will be injured, and if he isn't it is a miracle. There are proven, easy to learn and practice, techniques from Judo that will enable you to greatly reduce the chances of your being injured by a fall.

There are only three basic ways a person can fall: forward, backwards and sideways. Let us examine and practice techniques for each of these types of falls.

The Forward Fall: this particular fall has two basic techniques to it. One, when the athlete has enough momentum or room to do a forward roll; two, when he must fall straight down.

The Forward Roll: Practice methods. In this roll it is important to roll the shoulder over so that it does not hit the ground, and to have the same foot and same shoulder forward, i.e. your right foot and right shoulder. Tuck the chin, avoid supporting your weight with your wrist, keep the body in a ball, and continue your rolling momentum till your are standing up again.

Stages in learning - Beginning:

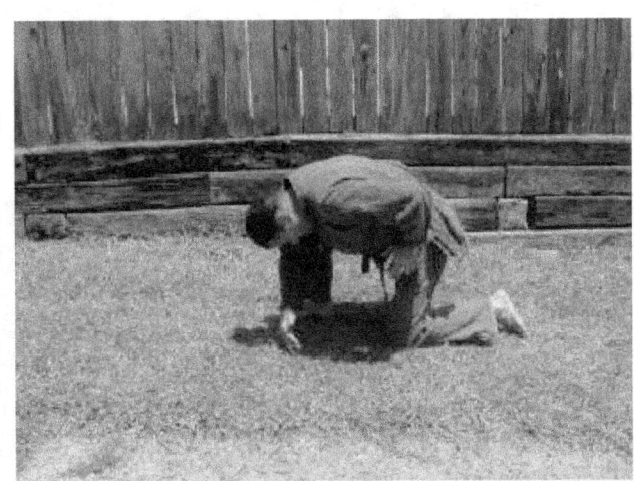

a. squat down with the right knee and right shoulder forward

b. lean over, tucking the head, and rolling the shoulder over forward

c. keep the body in a ball and land with one leg flat, the other straight ahead

d. roll up and stand.

Practice this at least 12 times from the right and left sides.

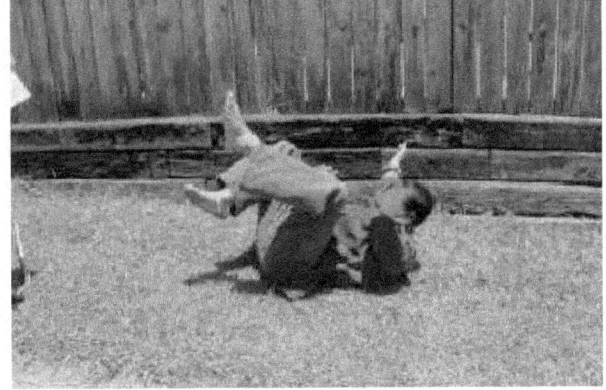

Intermediate Stage:

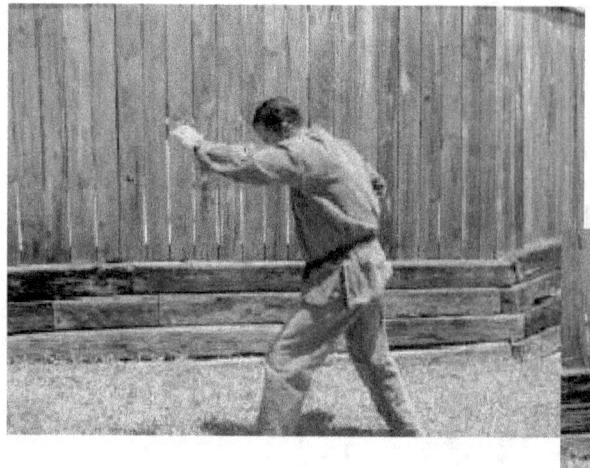

a. step forward with the right shoulder tucked down and the right leg forward

b. duck the head and bend over to the ground

c. curl the shoulder over and roll the body in a ball over the top of the shoulder

d. continue your roll till you are standing

Practice this roll at least 12 times with each shoulder. Be careful not to put too much weight on the wrist during the roll, and to tuck the head.

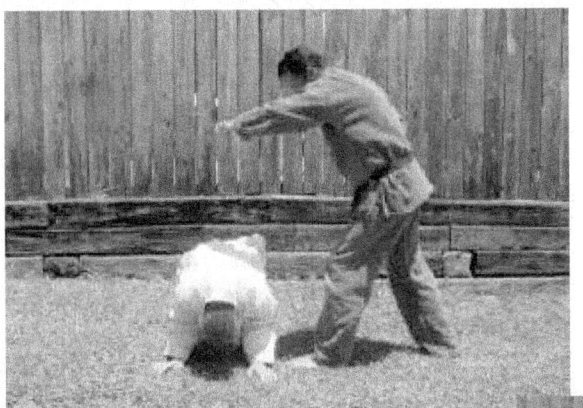

a. have one partner kneel on the ground, very low

b. take a running start and jump over the partner

c. while in the air tuck the shoulders and roll the body on the ground

d. continue the roll till you are standing up

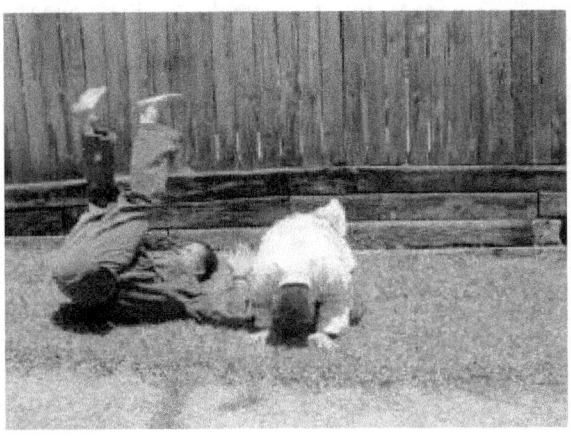

Continue to add people on the ground till you can jump over 5 people. Do this at least 12 times. Practice your intermediate rolls every day during your practice session and before a game. It helps warm up the body and get the blood circulating.

The Forward Break fall: sometimes the player will find that he is unable to do a forward roll because of a wall or other people, etc. Then it is necessary to do a forward break fall all to prevent injury. In this fall it is important to remember to absorb all the shock of the fall on the forearms and hands by slapping the ground very hard just before you hit it. Keep the head up and the back straight or slightly raised to keep the knees from hitting the ground.

Practice - Beginner:

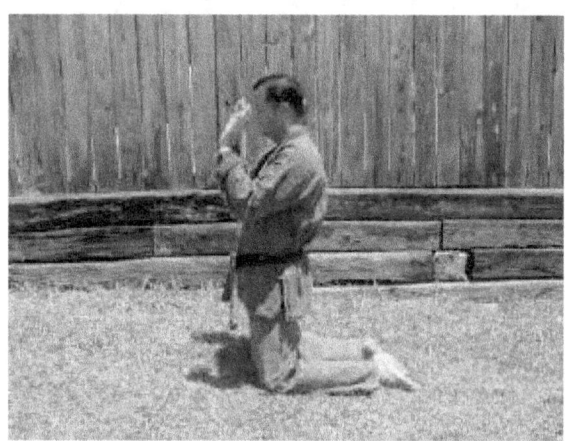

a. kneel on the ground with the hands in front of the body

b. fall forward slapping the ground very hard before you hit

c. keep the behind off the ground and the head up. Forcefully exhale your air as you hit

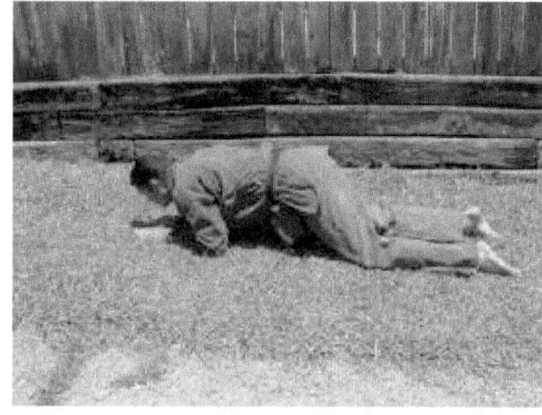

Practice this fall at least 12 times.

Intermediate:

a. stand up with the arms crossed in front of the body

b. bend the legs and slowly fall forward, slapping the ground very hard with the arms before hitting

c. keep the behind off the ground and the head up. Yell and let your air out as you hit.

Practice 12 times.

Advanced:

a. stand straight up with the arms by the sides

b. jump forward as far as you can, slapping the ground with the hands before you hit

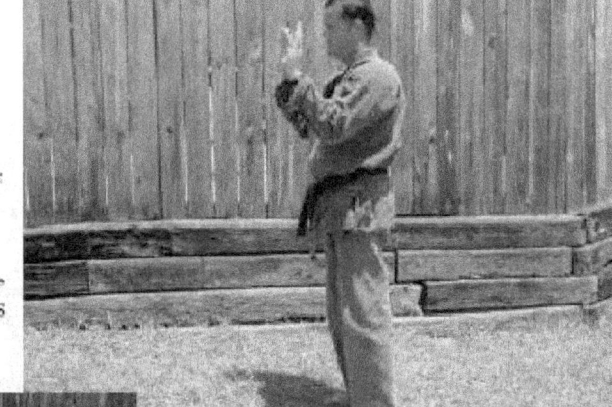

c. keep the trunk off the ground and the head up. Yell and forcefully exhale your air to keep it from getting knocked out

The Backwards Fall: often the player may find himself with his feet slipping out from under him or being knocked out from under him and must fall backwards without injuring his tail bone, or hitting his head.

The points to remember are to always bend the legs when slipping to get as close to the ground as possible before hitting, keep the chin tucked into the chest, slap with the arms as hard as you can, keeping the arms 45 degrees from the body, keep the back curved and the behind off the ground by slapping the ground before your butt hits it. Keep the legs crossed for protection, or to the sides.

Practice - Beginner:

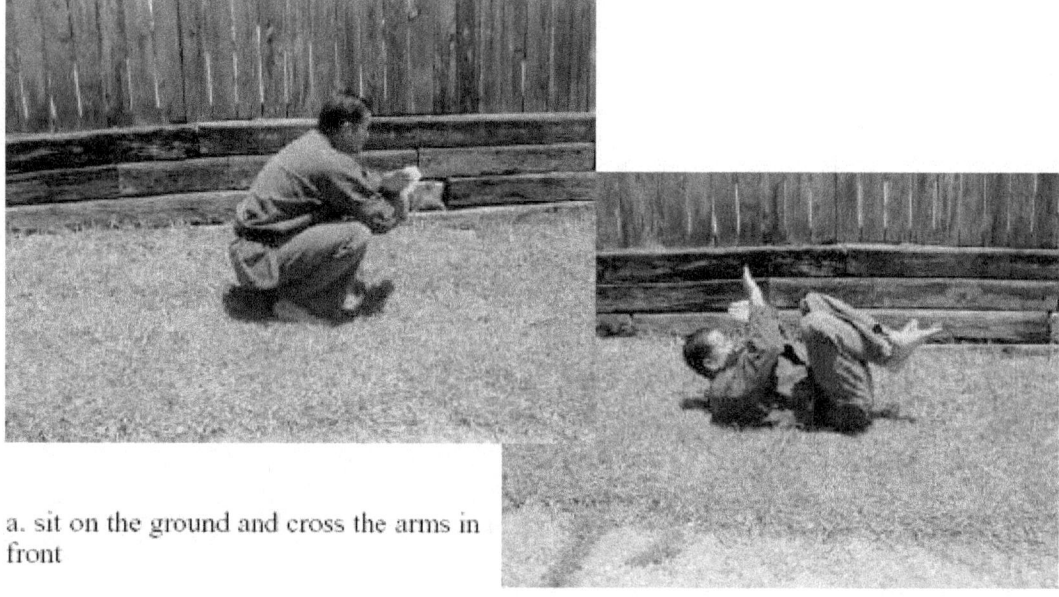

a. sit on the ground and cross the arms in front

b. slowly lean backwards slapping the ground very hard with the arms before your behind hits

c. keep the chin tucked into the chest, forcefully exhale the air

d. keep the back curved and the legs crossed or to the side

Practice this fall 12 times.

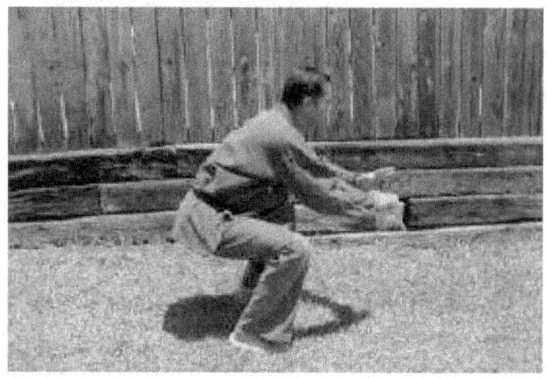

Intermediate:

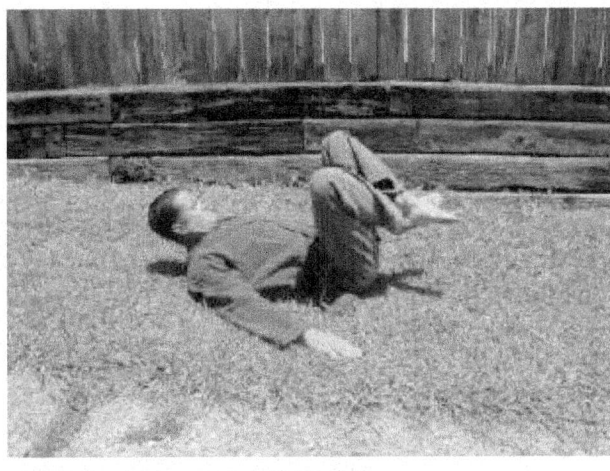

a. stand up with the arms crossed in front of the body

b. step backwards and begin to try to sit on the ground (an important point for it is much easier to fall from 1 foot than it is from 5 feet, and in most cases you are able to squat before you hit the ground.)

c. slap the ground very hard with the arms (notice how close the arms are to the body)

d. keep the butt off the ground until last, and the chin tucked into the chest so the head does not snap back and hit the ground. Yell to let your air out, so it does not get knocked out of you

Practice this fall 12 times.

Advanced:

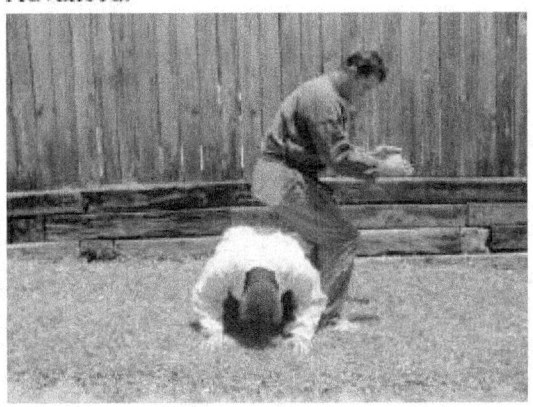

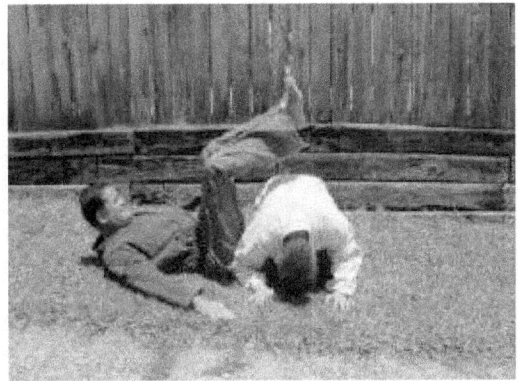

a. have a partner kneel on the ground very low

b. walk up briskly backward to the partner

c. fall over the partner and slap the ground before your butt or head hits, yell to let the air out so it does not get knocked out

d. continue to roll over and get back up

Practice this fall 12 times.

Note: the backwards fall is a very easy fall to take when one feels himself falling or has any type of warning he may be falling backwards. However, if one finds himself slipping on ice, etc., and falling backwards, then he must think very fast so as to avoid hitting his coccyx, or bumping his head. These fast reflexes come with practice.

The Side Break fall: often the player will find himself falling to the sides and care must be taken to avoid a shoulder injury or a wrist injury. The knee is particularly vulnerable in this position and proper falling and cover-up after falling can prevent many knee injuries.

The important points to remember:
- never try to break the fall with your wrist
- keep the legs straight, or the knees bent to avoid knee injuries during or after the fall
- slap the ground very hard
- exhale your air to keep it from being knocked out.

Practice - Beginners:

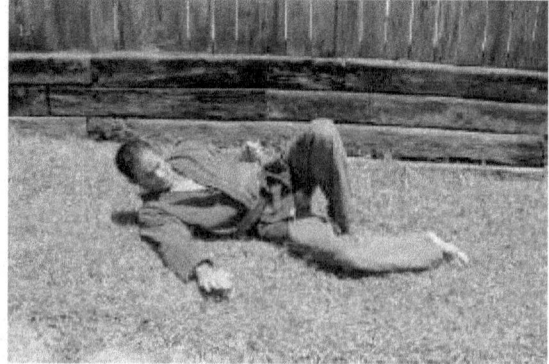

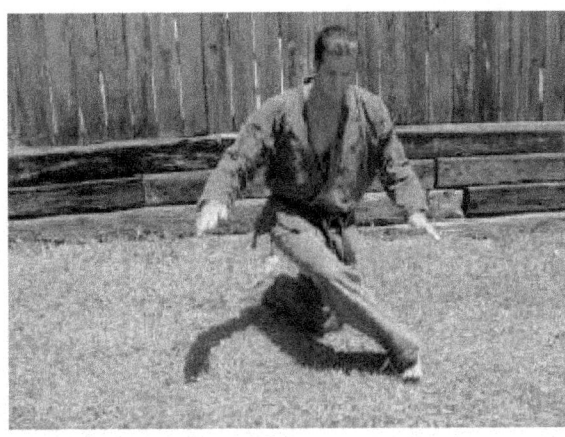

a. kneel on the ground with the right leg in front of the left leg

b. slowly let yourself fall to the right, slapping the ground very hard with the right arm (note distance of arm from body), keep the knees bent

c. keep the head off the ground

Practice this fall 12 times to each side

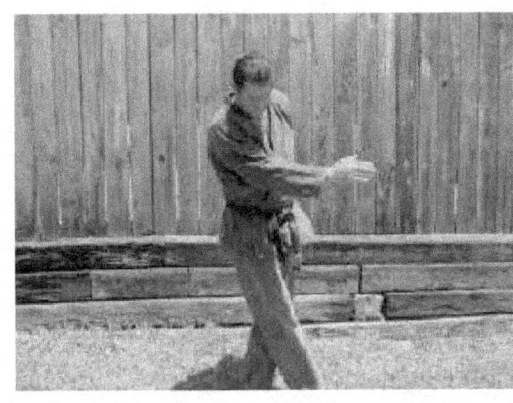

Intermediate:

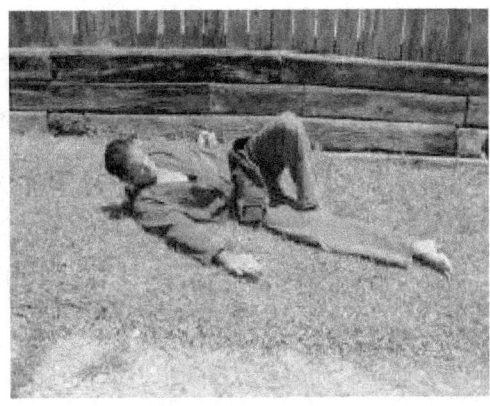

a. stand up with the right leg swinging across in front of the left.

b. slap the ground very hard before you hit, keep the shoulder curled forward

c. keep the knees bent

d. exhale your air forcefully to avoid having it knocked out

Practice this fall 12 times to each side.

Advanced:

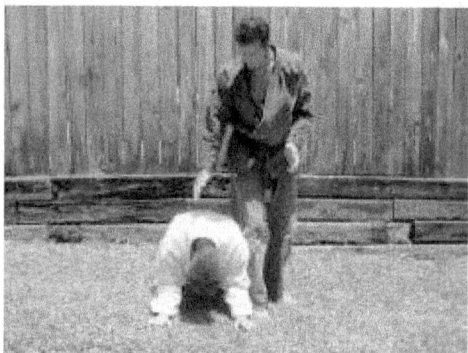

a. have a partner kneel on the ground

b. run up to the partner and jump over him landing on your side

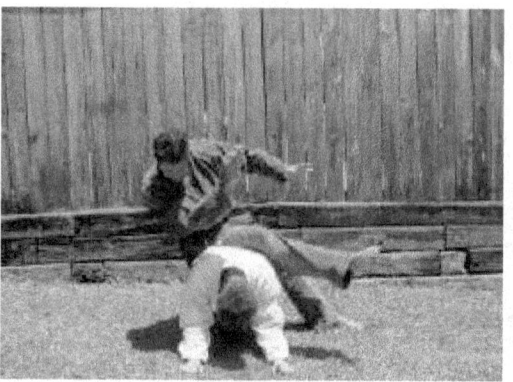

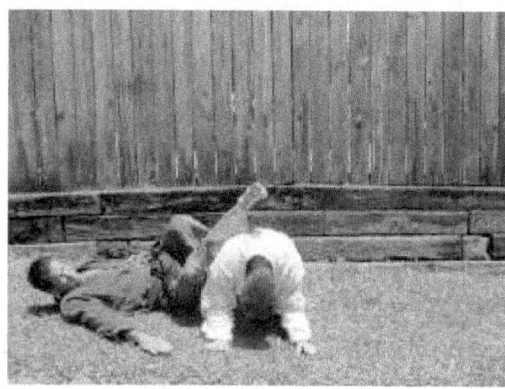

c. slap the ground very hard, yell, and keep the knees bent

Practice this fall 12 times to each side.

4 Way Falling Practice:

one of the best ways to practice your falls quickly and effectively.

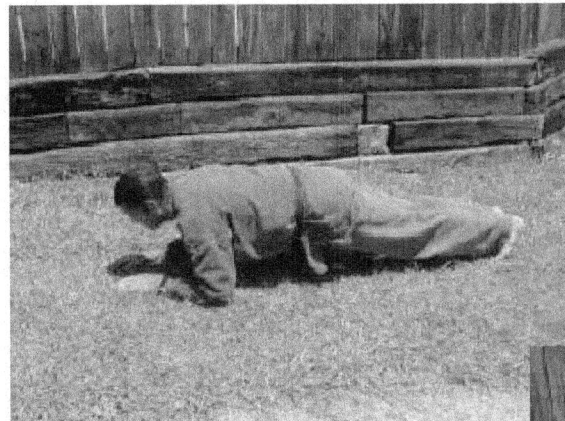

a. jump forward into the forward break fall, get up quickly

b. take a step and do a forward

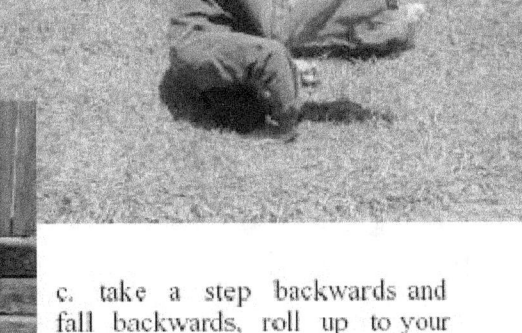

shoulder roll, roll up to your feet

c. take a step backwards and fall backwards, roll up to your feet

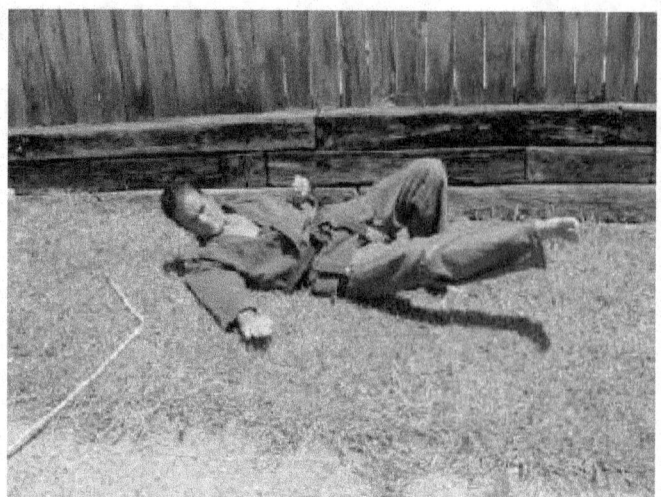

d. take a step sideways and fall to your side, cover and get up.

Do this 4 times alternating sides on applicable falls.

Falling: it is very important to practice these falls every day until you have mastered them to such an extent that they are second nature to you. Because in the real life situation you fall very fast and suddenly and you often only have a split second to think. Your reflexes must be sharpened to the extent that you can fall any direction with only the slightest notice. It may seem silly, but a good way to practice for these reflexes is to fall suddenly while you are walking, at your own discretion, and to practice and re-practice your falls especially the 4 way falling techniques till you have mastered them.

It seems that today despite the fact that there is better equipment, better playing fields, better and stronger athletes and better coaching, there are more knee injuries than ever before. I believe that is because the knee is usually not worried about until it is too late. Not nearly enough emphasis is put on techniques that could prevent a knee injury, and too much emphasis is placed on techniques that do little to prevent the injuries.

The knee can be injured in the same three ways any other body part can be injured. By falling down and tearing and pulling its tendons or ligaments, by over stretching the ligaments or tendons, and by getting hit and breaking it, tearing or stretching it too much. Three simple to do but effective techniques can be applied to help prevent most of the knee injuries.

Flexibility: it is important that the knee be flexible, but not to over stretch or tear the knee ligaments. So a simple rotary knee flexibility exercise is all that is needed. Bend slightly down and place both hands upon the knees. Make small circles to the right and to the left, about 10 in each direction. Now bounce up and down a few times and make 10 more circles to the right and left.

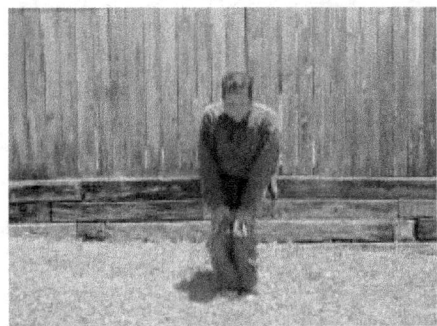 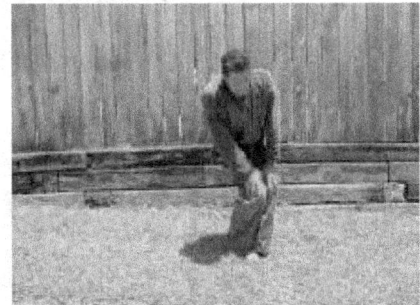

Ki in The Knee: The secret to not having the knee injured when you are hit in the knee is to have the knee bent into the blow. You can not be hit directly on the side or front of the knee. The knee must be slightly bent with the weight evenly displaced on both legs. As the blow comes you absorb most of the shock and control the knee in the direction you wish it to bend, not the direction he wants it to bend.

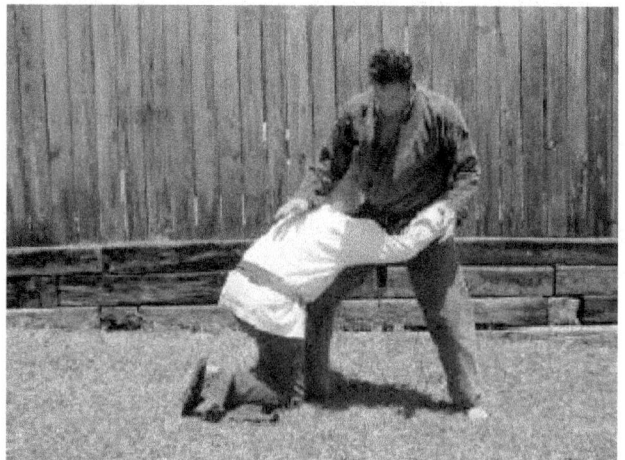

You can not take a blow directly on the front of the knee

a. stand with the feet slightly wider than shoulder width & the weight centered

b. have a partner get down beside you and push his body weight against the knees

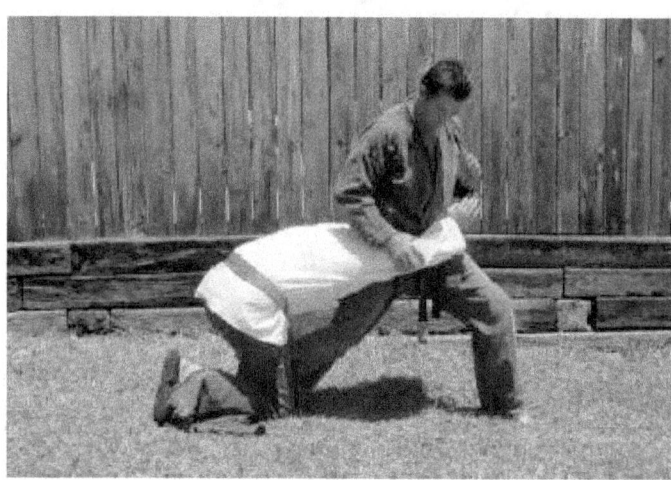

c. use your leg muscles to hold the knee tight and your breath control by breathing out very sharply to concentrate the muscles and control or focus the mind

65

d. shift your weight over to the opposite leg and begin to collapse forward with the knee being hit, bending the knee and consciously pulling it up to bend. Do not place a lot of weight on the ball of your foot so you can control the position of the fall.

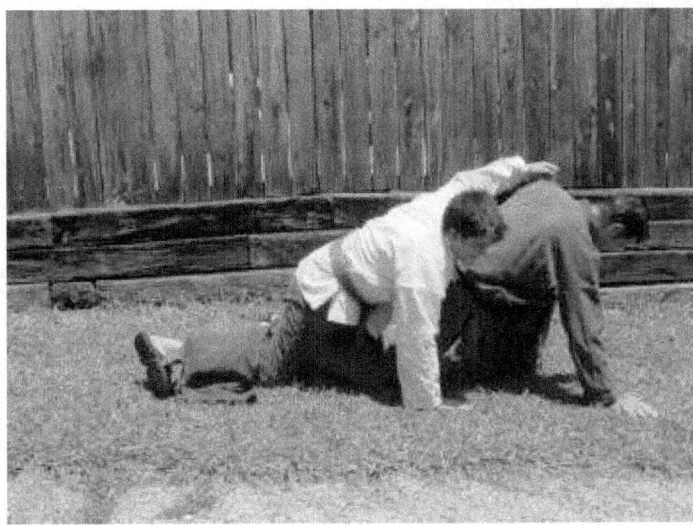

You must fold the knee into the direction of the hit

Falling to Protect The Knees: a simple rule to remember when you are hit on the knees or when you fall in any position to protect your knees. BEND THE KNEES and try to tuck them up, in other words fold your legs. You cannot have your knee injured if your legs are bent in half.

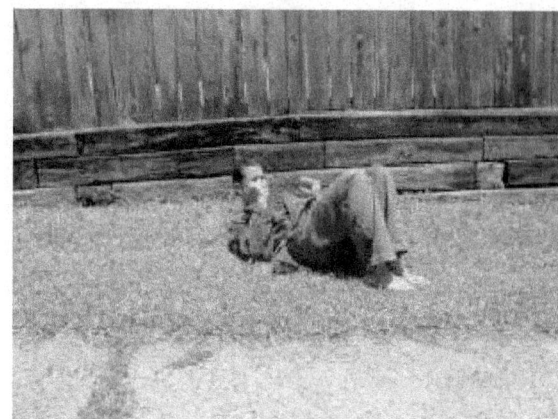

When falling in any position, bend the knees

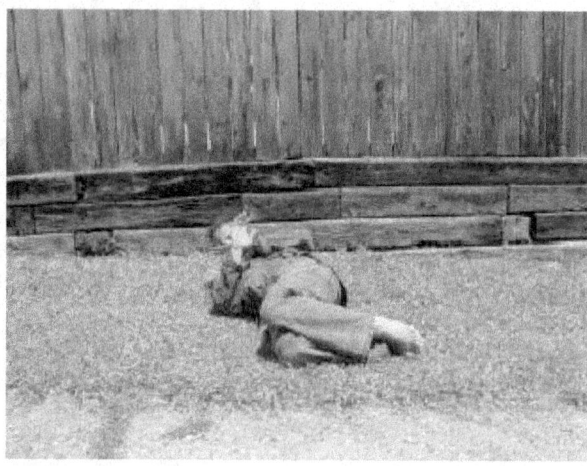

Sometimes the knee is injured after you have fallen because the leg is straight out on top of someone else and someone comes by and falls on it or steps on it and tears the knee. To avoid this think when you are on the ground the play is not over just because you are on the ground. When you are on the ground, immediately bend both knees up to your chest. If you find yourself with one leg out and caught so you can't bend it, then roll over on your stomach. If you can't bend your leg or roll over on your stomach, then try to lift the leg and bend it up.

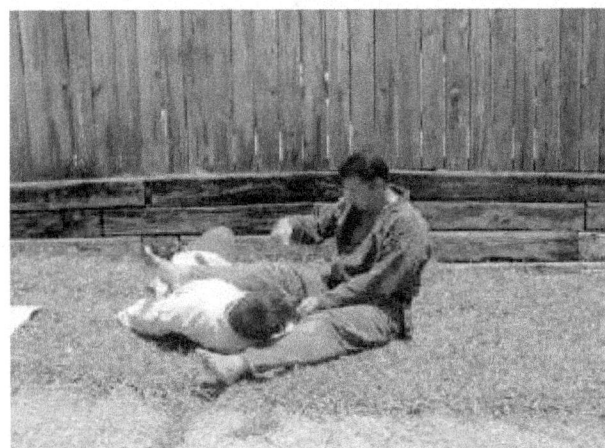

You must not lock the knee if it is on top of someone else.

Roll to the side and let the knee bend for protection

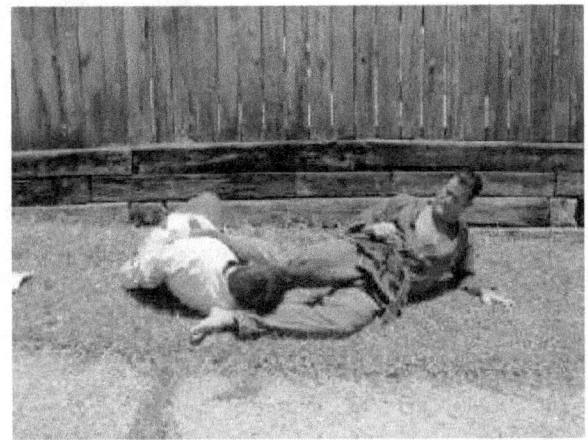

Remember the play is not over till the referee has the ball, you are in the huddle, or on the side line. Think when you are on the ground. Immediately take a look at your knees and bend them. **Bend them as quickly as you can or roll over.** Many times knee injuries could be prevented by this technique. Always remember to bend the leg up. Pull your body towards it.

RELAXATION

The ability to relax cannot be overemphasized and can be defined for our use to mean the ability to leave the game out of your body, but keep it in your mind. Too many coaches and players lose points, games and get ulcers because they cannot control their tempers or attitudes during the game situation. They have let their reactions be determined by the actions of other people, referees, or players. Therefore, they find themselves like puppets on a string, ranting and raving, or awkward and clumsy because they have destroyed the delicate relationship between the body and the mind. They have let their emotions take a disproportionate part in their actions and because of that they have lost their style, poise and grace. We have all seen far too many cases of this and know it's true. (For example: the coach in the ball game who runs up and down the side lines, kicking the ground and the players and screaming and shouting at the referee, the player who can't make a shot because he is so nervous and anxiety ridden, the player who jumps off sides several times or who starts fights for the slightest provocation.) The problem with these people is that they have lost control of their body by letting their mind become confused and disoriented. Your mind cannot think of two things at once and do a good job on either one. You must have a calm mind if you want to make the shot, or to think the play out. Your mind tells and directs your muscles to perform as they have been conditioned but if your mind is racing between being upset and making the shot, being angry and being relaxed then the muscles get contradictory information to them and subsequently do not perform as programmed but become un-coordinated. The brain becomes confused by the huge influx of emotional stimulus and can't reason intelligently, perform adequately and begins to send out all kinds of emergency signals to the body. You see, your mind cannot distinguish between a vividly imagined event and an actual occurrence. So when you begin to think angry, your brain interprets danger and sends out the appropriate body responses. Your adrenaline starts to be released, thereby causing the blood pressure to go up, the heart beats faster, the stomach stops digesting and begins secreting acid, the eyes dilate and the muscles become jerky and tensed. So your body is prepared for attack or defense and when none comes the damage is irreversible. No one is easier to handle than a drunk, or a man that has gone crazy and so angry that he is like a wild man, he obviously can't perform his primary function in the game and so your defense or offensive gets the advantage of having one more player on their side functioning at peak condition and one less on your side not only functioning poorly but probably causing others to perform badly. Ulcers and lost games, fights and lost friends are just some of the results of the inability to relax.

Any great athletic performance seems effortless because the athlete has practiced and practiced until he has programmed his body for the appropriate response. He has learned to keep his mind calm and to relax while performing, thereby conserving his energy and assuring a longer and better performance. He is like a work of art, graceful and beautiful to look at, because he has achieved harmony between his body and mind. A great coach is the same thing. He has learned to teach and train his team with patience, kindness and understanding. He has confidence in his team and his coaching staff. He knows that they will do the best that they can, and that the game is not the time to change previously conditioned responses or to try to do a coaching job that should have been done in practice sessions. So he remains calm and relaxed on the sidelines and usually winds up winning. Of course there are coaches who become involved to a great extent and are also winners, but they don't last as long and generally pay for their involvement with ulcers and loss of friends and support. No one likes you when you are upset especially your own body. So let's practice a form of relaxation that takes only 3 minutes and can be as beneficial as 1 hour of sleep.

Relaxation Technique: lie on the floor with the feet together and the palms face down on the sides of the body. Look straight up and do not move the eyes. This is important. Now take a deep breath, hold it for a second and tighten the feet. Now relax and exhale. As you do, say mentally to yourself, "relax, my feet are relaxed." Now take a deep breath and tighten the calves. old the tension a second. As you release the

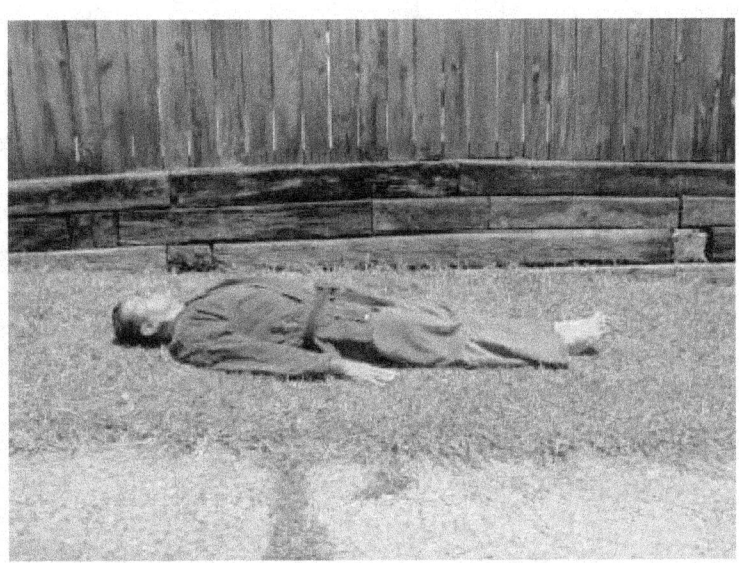

breath say gently to yourself "my calves are relaxed." Take another deep breath and tighten the thighs. Hold it for a second. As you release the breath, relax the thighs.

Your legs are now completely relaxed. You no longer wish to move your legs. You could move your legs, but you no longer wish to move them. Take a deep breath into your stomach, hold it. As the air leaves your stomach, relax your stomach. Now breathe deeply into your lungs. As the air leaves your lungs, relax your chest and let your breath become very subtle and soft. Now breathe and tighten the arms and hands. Hold the tension a second. Then relax. As the breath leaves your arms become very relaxed. Your entire body is now very relaxed and you feel as if you are floating on a cloud, very calm and very relaxed. Take a breath and tighten your neck and shoulders. Hold it and as you let your breath out relax your neck area. Now take a breath and make a large frown, an ugly face. Now relax and breathe out, and relax your face, more and more till your jaw almost drops open. Your entire body is now completely relaxed and you feel extremely calm and relaxed. The only thing left to relax are your eyes. Gently close your eyes. You should immediately start dreaming now.

Just let your mind roam and relax, dream of soft and nice things. Imagine you are floating on a raft in a calm lake, or sailing on a cloud. Relax and feel the air flow through your body, relax and dream. Relax and dream. Let the mind float from one thought to the next, paying no special attention to any thought. Just watch them come and go in the mind like you see cars come and go on the highway. Relax and think of beautiful things. Think of nature, music, art, of love. Relax and feel yourself floating.

Now when one wishes to come out of this relaxed atmosphere, one should not just jump up. Gently open the eyes and take a deep breath and move the fingertips and the toes, breathe again and move the arms and the legs, breathe again and bend the arms and legs, and move the hips. Now take the arms and rub the back of the neck and calmly sit up and relax in a meditative posture for a few more seconds. You will feel very relaxed and quite calm and refreshed. This is truly a valuable way of letting an athlete relax and should be used by all serious students.

Three minutes of this relaxation is better for the body than 1 hour of sleep because it calms the nerves, refreshes the spirit, and soothes the mind. It is fast and simple to do and can be used after a workout or running (three minutes of sitting on the side of the track with the head between the legs trying to regain the breath after running does very little to relax you, while three minutes of this exercise does wonders.)

You can do this exercise lying down and it is very helpful to those who have trouble going to sleep. You can also do this standing up or sitting down during the game on the sidelines. As a coach, just take a few deep

breaths and tighten the muscles just as if you were lying down. In a few breaths you will begin to become calm and feel more relaxed. Just close your eyes for a few seconds and suggest to yourself a few pleasant thoughts. Your mind should become calm and relaxed and subsequently your performance as a coach and player will be at its strongest point.

The mind cannot be relaxed and calm when the body is breathing fast and furiously. So the necessity of regaining control over your breath as soon as possible after exertion is very important. Often when we run, we begin to experience anoxia and we get too much blood pumping too much oxygen and lose the delicate balance between good and bad air in our bodies. So we must use our mind to control our breathing and slow our breathing to allow the oxygen, carbon dioxide stages to be equalized.

Deep Breathing, or Circular Breathing:

To be used when you find yourself breathing too fast after exercise or after you exert yourself to assure that your muscles are getting an adequate supply of air.

Stand with the feet shoulder width apart and touch the hands together in front of the body. Begin the breath very slowly and easily as the arms are lifted up in a clockwise circle around the head and down the sides of the body, continuing to breathe in air the entire circle. Do this three times and one will feel much more refreshed and have a much more adequate air supply to necessary muscles. As you practice doing this exercise, you will learn to control your breathing and be able to get more benefit from the circular breathing. It is the fastest and easiest way to regain the proper breathing control after running or strong physical exertion.

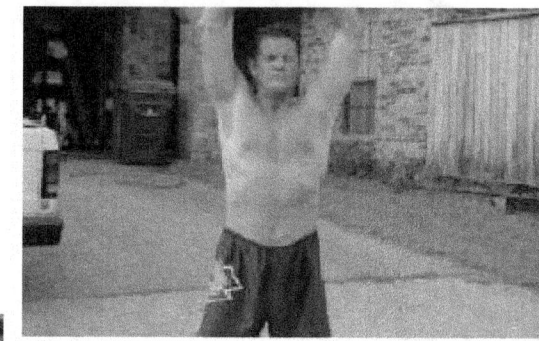

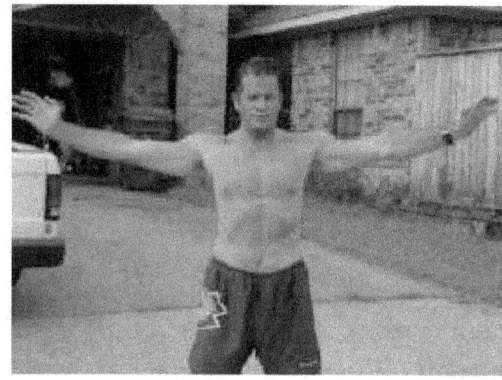

Raise the arms above the head and as you pull the arms down around your body, breathe in very deeply.

As you continue your circle breath out and you bring your arms back up to the top.

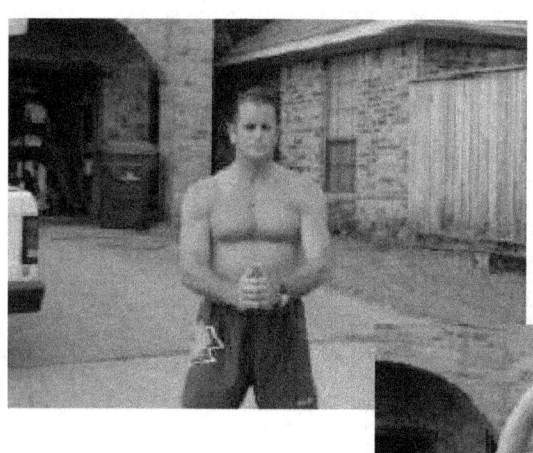

BREATHING EXERCISES

The breath plays a most important part in the relaxing of the body and often it is the breath that is the determiner of the body's responses, not the body that is determining the breath's reaction. In other words you are not breathing fast because you have been running, you are able to run because you are able to breathe quickly and supply the additional oxygen requirements to the body. You could not run at all if you could not breathe at all. In fact, you could not do anything at all if you could not breathe well. You would be asthmatic and unable to perform any vigorous exercise or to exert too much.

Your breath is the most important thing in your body. It is the only thing that you can not consciously deprive yourself of. You can poke your eyes out, kill yourself for love, bust your ear drums listening to loud music, deprive yourself of food, but you cannot hold your breath till you suffocate and you cannot let someone else suffocate you. Your body will not just relax and let itself be deprived of air. You will do anything to anyone when the need for air becomes dire for your survival.

The breath plays a very important part in relaxation because it plays a large part in the control of our body's reactions to certain events. For example, we have already noted that we could not run if we were not able to breathe fast and deep enough to supply the additional oxygen requirement needed by the body. When we are angry our breath becomes short and fast like when we are running. But when we are sleeping, our breath becomes slow and deep and relaxed and so is our mind. We cannot be breathing slow and deep and relaxed if we are angry. Just as we cannot be breathing slow and easy when we are upset. We breathe calm and our mind responds calmly, our muscles respond calmly. Your breath stills the mind and calms the nerves. So exercises have been developed centuries ago by people who understood the importance of the breath as a factor in self understanding and mind and body control. We will practice or study by practice, three of these methods.

Counting the Breaths: Sit in a meditative posture (see Chapter 10) and take a few deep breaths to calm the mind. Now begin to concentrate only on the breath as it comes in and as it leave the body. Try to clear the mind of all outside thoughts and concentrate only on the incoming and outgoing breaths. When you begin to breathe in, think only of the number One or only of this being your first breath. Let no other thoughts enter your mind but the number One. Continue to concentrate on this number all the way through the breath and as you begin to breathe out, continue to think and concentrate only on the number One. Now as you begin your next breath think and concentrate only on the number Two. Clear the mind of all other thoughts and think only of the number Two as you breathe in and as your breathe out. Continue to do this slow breathing and concentration up to the number Ten striving to keep the mind calm, not tense, and concentrating only on the numbers.

In a very few seconds you will see the extreme difficulty of clearing the mind and in only concentrating on the numbers. Thoughts will begin to float up and your mind will notice them and you will begin to feel and think about these thoughts and so become distracted from your primary purpose of thinking and seeing only the numbers. But do not become discouraged. This is an exercise and technique that can take literally years of practice to do perfectly. The mind is always full of extra thoughts and you must practice trying to calm it just as you would practice trying to learn a new skill, over and over again with patience and a calm and resolved manner. You cannot still the mind by being angry at it for thinking other thoughts, or calm the mind by tightening the muscles. Just relax and try to concentrate the mind only on the breath. Gradually you will be able to think only of the numbers.

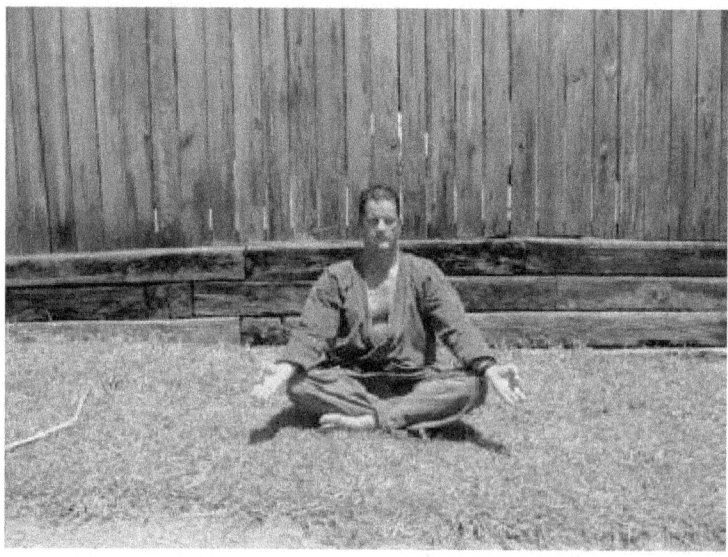

Counting The Breath 2. If you are having great difficulty in visualizing the numbers then perhaps the visualization of colors will be easier for you. when you breathe in, think only of the color red, through the entire breath, and then of the color blue, then green, then orange, then black, then white, then yellow, then brown, then purple, and finally pink, (or you can use any color you wish). This may be easier for you and provides a more pleasing visual stimulus for the mind.

You should perform this counting exercise every day for at least a few weeks until you have begun to gain some mastery over your mind and some control of your mind. Practice should only take a few minutes, up to five, and so should not be troublesome to you for finding the time to practice. After you have begun to get good in this you may want to do it more often for the relaxing effects it has on the mind and body. You may do it as often or as little as you wish. You can do it on the sidelines when you find yourself getting upset (remember how your mother told you to count to ten if you were angry). The same effect is achieved now but you are adding the effect of the slow and easy breathing to calm the nerves and soothe the mind.

Controlling The Breath: this exercise trains one in the voluntary control of the breath by the conscious will of the mind. You will not be allowing the body to breathe normally but will be trying to force it to breathe as the mind wishes.
Sit in the meditative posture and close the eyes. Take a few deep breaths to calm the mind and now slowly begin to breathe in for the count of 10, count each number silently to yourself. Now hold your breath without pressing down or lifting your shoulders up for the count of 10. Now begin to breathe out for the count of 10, trying to make the out-breathing slow and controlled and not breathe out all the air at the beginning of the out-breath. Immediately after you have breathed out for 10, begin to breathe in again for the count of 10. Hold it for 10 and out for 10. Do this exercise 10 times. You will find that you may start to sweat and that you really have to use a lot of muscles and mind control to stop your body from breathing in too quickly or out too fast. This is an excellent form of breathing control and the benefits are numerous. It teaches the mind great strength and begins to reconfirm to the muscles the power of the mind over them. It produces a body heat, and so can be used if you are cold; and it strengthens the breath control by the actual controlling g of the breathing movement. You can consider yourself exceptional if you can breathe in for 30 seconds, hold it for 30 seconds and breathe out for 30 seconds - 10 times. This shows a true mastery of the breath and a great deal of muscle and mind control. Do this exercise daily for a few weeks until you have been able to do all ten breaths in the correct count. Thereafter you may do it as often as you wish for the benefits to the muscles, the body and the mind.

Following The Breath: the purpose of this exercise is to transcend the mind and to concentrate only on the breath as it fills the body and the lungs and to follow it as it comes and goes in and out. This is a very soothing and relaxing form of breathing and the benefits are long lasting and comforting.

Sit in the meditative posture, close the eyes and take a few deep breaths to calm the mind and relax the nerves. Now as you begin to breathe in, try to let all other thoughts leave the mind except following the breath as it goes through your nostrils, down your throat and fills your lungs, then is dispersed to the various parts of your body. Follow it as it returns up your throat and out your nostrils and into the air. Try to imagine a golden string being attached to your lungs that comes out of you as you breathe the air out and comes back into the lungs as you breathe in. Let your mind remain calm and follow the breath softly and easily. Soon you will begin to feel the body become filled with air and begin to feel very calm and relaxed, very soothed and light. The breath will fill your mind and your body and you will begin to feel as light as your breath itself. Do this exercise as long as you feel light and are able to concentrate on following the breaths. It is very soothing and relaxing. Perform this exercise any time you are upset or any time you wish to feel truly relax

THE TIGER EYE

The "Tiger Eye" is a term that we will use to mean peripheral vision, or the ability to see everything that is surrounding you without the necessity of moving the eyes or the head. This technique is very valuable in most sports and causes an increase in awareness and subsequently performance. If you can see everything that surrounds you, the chances of your throwing an interception, or missing a tackle or shot are greatly reduced.

The Meditative Position: there are as many different positions for meditation (or concentration on a specific thought towards a specified goal) as there are forms of meditation. All have their benefits but some of them are difficult to get into position to do. So we will use a simple but effective position, called in Yoga the half lotus position.

Sit on the floor with the legs crossed in front of the body. Place the right leg in first and cross the left leg in front of that. Strive to keep the knees as near the ground as possible and the back, spine and neck in a straight line. Rock back and forth and gently to the sides to assure you are sitting up straight. Place the arms on the tops of the knees with the palms up. This helps to stabilize and balance the back. You may feel uncomfortable in this position. That is because you are not flexible enough. To improve flexibility do the stretches found in the front of the book, but if you are not flexible because you have not been doing the stretches long enough you may modify the position so that you are grabbing the knees or even putting the legs straight out. You may even sit in a straight backed chair while you are learning your flexibility.

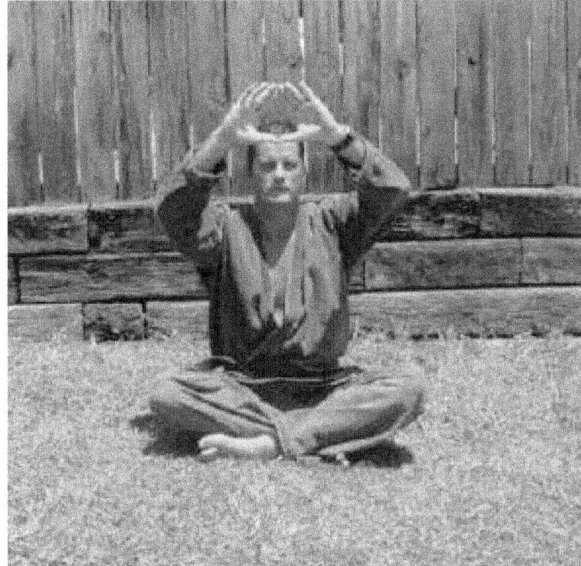

The half lotus position. Note the straight back, the arms on the knees, the left leg in front of the right, and the steady and calm eyes.

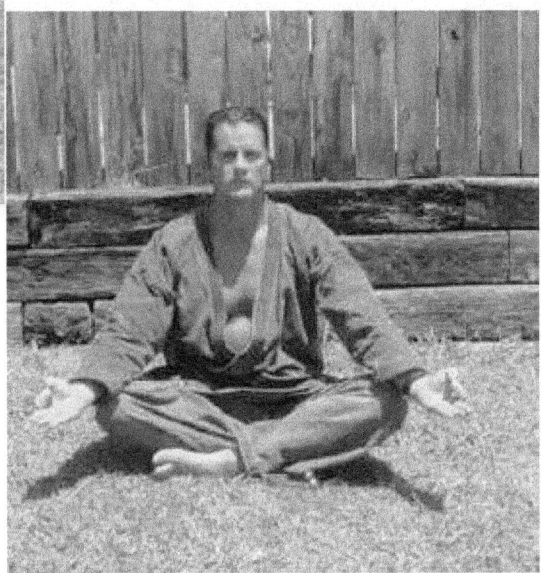

One should sit in the half lotus position while practicing the Tiger Eye and the gaze should be straight ahead with the eyes not moving to fix a point for the gaze.

The hands should be held above the head to start with, the fingers forming a triangle, and then slowly brought down to in front of the eyes. There the eyes should be fixed in their gaze upon one area and no longer move. The hands should then be placed on the knees, palms up with the thumb and forefinger inter joined. Now the Tiger Eye should be practiced.

After one has assumed the meditative posture one should fix the gaze of his eyes directly ahead and on one point. Let us assume you are looking at a football field during a game and you are standing in the middle of the field facing the goal line. Now without moving your eyes you can see the following things. You can see the goal posts and the end zone. You can see the stripes on the field and the grass, and the colors of the grass. You can see the sidelines, and the benches full of other players on the sidelines. You can see the players on the playing field, all of the players, and you can see the sky. You can see the lights around the stadium and the fans in the seats around the stadium. You can see the players directly beside you and across from you. In other words, you can see everything - in front of you, on the side of you, above you, and below your feet.

Now listen, you can hear the crowd. You can hear the sports announcer. You can hear the coach and players yelling on the sidelines. You can hear the quarterback and the players on the field talking, and even walking or hitting each other on the plays. You can see everything and you can hear everything going on around you. This is total awareness, total visual and sensory awareness. You cannot be surprised by a clip, or scared by a yell of another player. You are aware, just like the tiger is aware in the jungle. Yet you are relaxed and ready to move in any direction at any time, just like the tiger in the jungle.

You will find upon investigation that when the eyes are looking straight ahead and not focusing too sharply on one particular object that all the field of vision can be seen. But if you move your eyes side to side very fast or move your head quickly, then everything becomes blurred and you can actually not see things clearly. Just like a good hunter only looks at the trees and notices the slightest movement, not at the individual limbs and sees only that limb. Just imagine that the field is like a small painting. You can see all of the painting clearly but not if you are moving your head from side to side or your eyes quickly from side to side. So try to get in the habit of moving the whole body when you move the eyes. That way you are always keeping the vision clear and the body in such a position to react accordingly and effectively. (for example, if you look out the corner of your eye, you can see. But if someone was going to hit you and you could just see him in the corner of your eye, your body would not be in a very strong position for defending yourself. It is better to turn the whole body to look.) before, and you will thus be practicing your peripheral vision and soothing the nerves and calming the mind. The more you become aware of the things around you, the more you begin to appreciate them and their beauty.

The "Tiger Eye" is most useful for foul shooting, quarterbacks, safeties, and linebackers and for coaching (for all good coaches are able to look at the play and see the whole play unfolding at once, not just one player at a time. So a spotter who uses this technique will be a more effective spotter because he will be able to see the whole field and whole play at once.)

The "Tiger Eye" also involves listening for when you are relaxed and noticing all the sights around you, you are also noticing all the sounds around you. A good player is not drawn off sides by the change in the quarterback's cadence or inflection, and a good player does not lose concentration when the crowd boos him or is screaming at him or the team. He is just concentrating on the shot, or the game. He hears the noise but is not distracted by it.

You can practice the Tiger Eye while walking around school or at home. Just look straight ahead when you walk and do not move the eyes. You will see all the people coming and going around you and any movement to the right and left. You will feel calm and hear things you have not noticed

VISUALIZATIONS

Visualization is the conscious action of forming mental pictures in the mind. These pictures can be used for learning, for relaxation and for improvement of skill of techniques. We shall discuss techniques for doing these things.

Learning Through Visualizations: As we have noted previously the mind interprets and integrates the thoughts or sensations that occur and translates them into visual concepts or pictures inside the mind. These pictures formed in the mind are unable to be differentiated in the mind as being true or just products of the mind itself. In other words the mind cannot distinguish between a vividly imagined event and an actual occurrence. Therefore the mind can be programmed to believe certain concepts and ideas and when the mind internalizes or really believes these concepts the body will tend to find ways to make them come true. (for example, if you constantly believe you will be an All American, your body will be given the mental determination necessary to achieve the physical skills necessary to become an All American.)

The body cannot perform any skill that the mind cannot clearly see the body already being able to perform in intricate detail. You cannot be a great tennis player if you cannot see yourself making great tennis shots in your mind. I do not mean see the great shot (the ball being hit very fast or to the corner). You must be able to see every muscular position of your body in every aspect that you would be in if you are actually making the great shot.

If we would like to use visualization for learning, let us say for learning a new play in football, we can use the following exercises:

Meditation Imagination: sitting in the meditative posture, close the eyes and imagine you are about to perform the play which you are trying to learn. Where are your feet supposed to be as you come up and get down on the line? Who is to the right of you, the left of you, who is across from you, where are you supposed to make him go, or block him to? What noises will you be hearing at the start of the play? At the snap of the ball what is the first movement of your feet, where are your shoulders and arms supposed to be, who is beside you now, and what is the new position of the man facing you? As you move toward him, how are your feet supposed to be, what is his movement, where is the ball carrier? What noises are surrounding you, as you make contact where are your arms and legs supposed to be, how far back and to what direction are you supposed to move him? Take yourself in your mind step by intricate step through the entire play. Do this several times, each time adding new points to your movement or blocking that you may have forgotten before. This is an excellent and effective way to practice and learn new plays, or improve on old ones. You can do this at home, while lying in bed, or while walking, or in the classroom.

Written Learning: have the student write down on a piece of paper all the various aspects of the play. What his job is, where he is supposed to be at the snap, at the first movement, who is he blocking and to where, for how long, who is beside him, to the right and left? When is the ball snapped and how long does the play last? Have him write down in intricate detail the entire play and read it to you or the group tomorrow for group discussion. Then tell him points he left out or that could be improved. He will be using techniques of visualization at home when he writes this down, as he uses the mind to organize and picture the entire play.

Coaching Learning: have the player take you through the play step by step, as if he were the coach. You take his place in the line and make the same mistakes and errors he previously made, or new ones to see how he can correct you, and those around him. You learn more by teaching than you do by playing and by letting him coach you he will be learning the play from teaching. He will have to visualize in his mind and tell you what you are doing wrong or right and so be reinforcing the learning.

Visualization of A Winner: It is not enough to say "We are number 1" and repeat it over and over if the player and the coaches really cannot see themselves as being number 1. because they cannot see themselves beating the tough teams. So if you would want to use visualizations to get the mind to really believe that you can beat the tough teams and that you can be number 1 practice the following exercise.

Assume the meditative posture and close the eyes. Now vividly imagine that you are at the ball park just as the game is about to be over with your toughest rival. Use all your senses in the visualization. Hear the roar of the crowd, smell the air, feel your uniform on your back and your muscles after a hard game, touch the ground and the players around you, taste the sweat dripping down your forehead from a hard fought battle. See the field and the scoreboard and see your team ahead with just one minute to go. Begin to watch the clock as you see the other team hopelessly trying to stop your drive, but it's too late because you have 3 downs left and they have no timeouts. Count the seconds down on the clock as you listen to the fans begin to count with you. Feel the excitement in the air, smell the excitement, begin to get excited and jump up and down, shaking hands and slapping the backs of the other players. At last, the clock is down to 10 seconds and the crowd is starting to gather around the field, 3, 2, 1, bang! The game is over and you jump for joy. You have beaten the best team in the league. Now you can really hold up your finger and say we are number. Vividly imagine this every night before you go to sleep, practice it as a team months before the big game, internalize the belief and use the visualization again and again. Your mind will come to believe it and accept it as a true fact, and the body will have the desire and determination to practice and the courage and skill to keep on trying and not make any mistakes in the big game and so assure the victory that you have by now become confident of in your mind.

Visualizations for Relaxation: have you ever been to the Alps, or Europe, or the Queens castles in England, or the Amazon in Brazil? Probably not, but in your mind you have because of the wonders of TV and movies. You have formed visual pictures of these places in your mind and it is just like you were really there. The ability to form these visual pictures can be used as a form of relaxation before sleep or to help you go to sleep and have pleasant dreams. Lie down and take a few deep breaths to calm the mind, now slowly let your mind drift over some pleasant thoughts and scenes like the mountains, the lakes, or the forest. As one of these thoughts begins to get clear in the mind, softly begin to linger there and to visualize yourself standing in the middle of the mountain beauty, feel the soft breeze on your face, and smell the clean fresh air. Look around you at the wonders of nature, and hear the beautiful sounds of life that surround you. Begin to hear soft and lovely music as you continue to enjoy the sights. Perhaps now

you have been joined by a loved one you miss and would love to be sharing this scene with. Talk to them as if they were there and touch and feel them as if they were there. Let your mind float and your thoughts expand with the scenery until in your mind you feel as though you were really there. After a few minutes you will become very calm and relaxed and begin to truly dream or sleep.

Chapter 12

GOAL SETTING

The art of goal setting to many people is often confused as day dreaming because they have hazy goals, or goals that are unrealistic for them to achieve in the foreseeable future. Such things as being a millionaire, owning a mansion, or being President. You can be all things if you believe in yourself, develop a sensible and workable plan for achieving the results you desire, and have such a burning desire and determination to achieve your goals that no one or no thing will stop you. Goals to us will not mean far off day dreams. Goals are plans, feasible and workable plans, that are actively being pursued in an organized and predetermined fashion.

Why is it necessary to have goals, you might be saying. Well suppose you had a child and you wanted to teach him to throw and catch a baseball. That is your goal or your plan. In order to do it in the most effective and fastest way, it is logical that you develop his skills little by little and have a purpose in each thing you show him as a development of the skill of throwing and catching a baseball. He can't throw the ball with either hand, he must specialize and practice on just one, and he can't just throw the ball up, or backwards he must throw it towards a target. He must have a target to aim at and the reward comes when he hits his target. If you just give the child a ball and say go and play, he will develop improper or inadequate skills and usually become frustrated and give up on the sport. But if you have a plan for teaching him the skills and time for him to practice the skills then the goal of throwing a baseball is achieved in the fastest time and with the most effective of results.

The same thing is true of an athlete. He can't just have a vague goal or no goal at all and just want to play football. He must have a definite position that he must learn to play, he must have definite skills he must acquire in order to excel at that position and he must have a plan of action for achieving or practicing these skills that he will be learning. If he just goes out and tries every position and never learns or practices the skills necessary to excel in that position, he is a man without goals, or plans he is actively working on, and will get nowhere in football or life.

Everyone has goals they are working on. Unfortunately most people are working towards someone else's goals. Especially in sports too many players are just working on the goals the coaches have for them to achieve. They are lucky if the coach has a plan for them to be number one that is specifically outlined, and not just a slogan "We're number 1" on the wall. So they go through their careers never achieving the potential greatness within themselves. If the player would make it his goal to become an All American and map out in intricate detail the problems he has to overcome, the solutions to these problems, the time he has to achieve his goal and the progressive steps in achieving them, then there is no reason he cannot become an All American.

Some of the things the player should take into consideration in his becoming an All American are: How fast does he have to be able to run to be an All American? What should his muscular strength be? How much time should he practice a day, and on what skills? How many blocks, tackles, assists, etc., will he need to make in a game? How many yards will he need to gain, or stop the other team from gaining? Does he need the cooperation of other players or the coaches? How many seasons does he have left to play and when can he realistically expect to make the All American Team? What special skills does he have to achieve to be All American?

These and other questions must be answered by the player in detail before he begins his quest for becoming an All American. After he has answered these questions he must now begin to write a plan of action, for practice time, coaching time, weight training time, study time, etc. He must write down and organize himself to the smallest detail for what he needs to achieve and when he will practice to achieve these goals each day. Then he must begin working on his plan, every day without fail, determined and persistent in the pursuit of his goal. If the player remains resolved and keeps his vigorous practice schedule up, there is no reason he cannot make All District, All State and then All American.

The coaches should also have goals and intricate plans of action for the production of the skills they want the members of the team to have. Such things as: How many players should be able to bench 300 lbs. and run the 40 in 4 seconds? How many players of each position should they pursue in recruitment? How many victories do they need to win the conference? How many fumbles would be acceptable each game? (I know none is desired but what is the limit) How many yards should the offense gain, the defense let happen? How many field goals should they get in each specific game? How many touchdowns should they get in each game? How many points should they get? How many points should each player get? What does the asst. coach expect from each player? What does the coach expect from each asst. coach?

These and many many other questions the coaches should ask themselves and answer in detail so they know exactly what they have to get in each game and from each player and under what situations. If they are not sure of certain points they should make it a point to find out exactly what they expect at every possible time and event. Then the coach should write a plan of action and begin to follow it religiously day by day, hour by hour. His time should be devoted to and organized such that he is always making definite progress for his personal and team goals.

Practicing: often the optimal effects are not achieved during the practice session for many various reasons, but every practice session can be extremely productive and rewarding if the players and coaches can learn to relate to this story.

The Japanese women's volleyball team practices 365 days a year, 3 hours a day, and the women are never heard to complain or ever miss a practice. Each practice session is done as if it were before the big game and each player gives 110% each time they practice. That is why they are number 1 in the world. But what attitudes are in the minds of the women as they practice? The answer may surprise you. If you were to walk up to one of the girls and ask her, "How long have you been practicing, when do you get a break, why don't you get a day off?" or any of a dozen other questions that seem to fill the minds of the press and the fans. The answer would be, "I'll be right with you, right now I am playing volleyball." Not "I have been playing for 234 days without a break, I am sick of playing, the coach is mean, I never get a day off, I have been playing 2 hours and only have an hour to go, thank God". But just "I am playing volleyball." You see, the Japanese women have learned to master the art of concentration and because of that their mind is only on the game of volleyball, only on the point at hand not on yesterday's mistakes, tomorrow's practice, or next year's practice.

Not on the coach, but only on the game at that very minute. Extreme, intense, complete concentration on the present moment, at one specific thing. To make the point. Now! So in your practice session, or your game, your mind should not be wandering on when session will be over, or on the last play, or on how big the guy is you're trying to block or tackle, or on how many games you have left, or on your girl friend. You should play one play at a time and use all your concentration and energy and skill to do what you are supposed to be doing in that one particular play. Block that guy, tackle that guy, throw to that guy, only concentrate on that one fact. If you blow it, forget it and begin to concentrate on the next play, and your next block. Make one play at a time, one tackle at a time, and keep your mind concentrated just like the volleyball team.

Chapter 13

HOW TO DEVELOP EXPLOSIVE POWER IN YOUR MOVEMENT

No other sport in the world generates as much explosive power through movement as does Karate. Weight lifters have a lot of strength, but not the kind that makes for speed and agility, combined with power. Karate has developed techniques that enable people of slight build and small muscle mass to hit so hard and kick so powerfully that they are able to smash through bricks, wood or bodies. How do they get that power and how can you get it? By simply practicing the following exercises:

Hip Movement: most athletes use only the strength of one muscle part. In other words, a boxer hits you with his arms, a weight lifter pushes with his legs or arms, a football player hits you with his elbow or shoulder. They have not learned the tremendous amount of power that can be generated by the use of the entire body, especially the snapping and thrusting of the hips, to generate explosive power. Muscle alone will not be enough power. Imagine a very heavy sledge hammer. The power potential is enormous, but it is so heavy that you cannot swing it with enough speed to generate any force or power. So the huge potential power of the sledge hammer is essentially wasted.

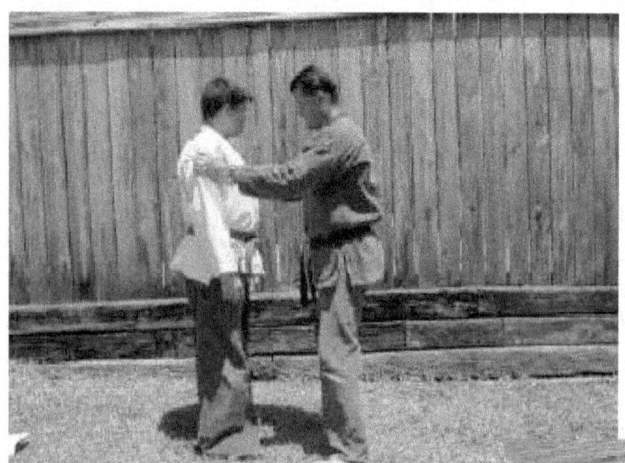

The same is true of many athletes. They have tremendous potential for power but they are too slow or do not use but one body part to generate this power and so reduce their effectiveness many times. The power that can be generated by a body is equal to this formula: $P = S \times M \times BM$ or Power equals Speed of the movement times the muscular strength behind it times the unified body movement at the time of impact. So we must work to develop speed, coordination and muscle and use all three simultaneously and focus them at the point and instant of contact.

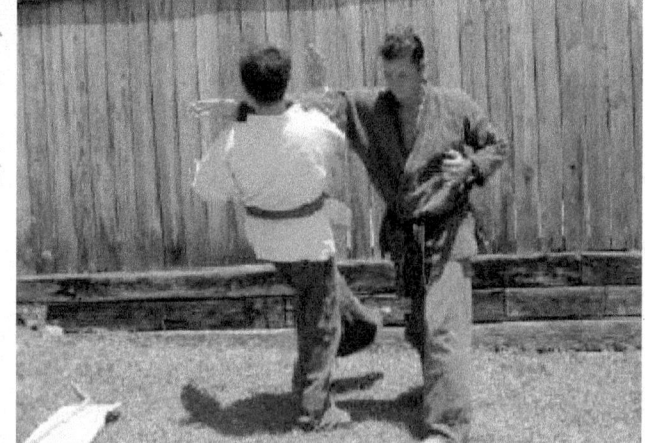

Weight Shifting Exercise: have the partners stand facing each other with the arms on the shoulder of one partner. Now without moving his arms any wider than they already are, one partner must generate a whipping action of the hips and throw the partner to the side. Upon trying to do this, it is easy to see that if one tries to throw him to the side with just his arm strength, he cannot do it. Do this at least 15 times with each partner and practice every day until mastered.

One Inch Punch: using the hips as a power generator and locking the arm in the manner we have learned from the unbendable arm techniques one can develop devastating power from only one inch away from the partner.

Have the partners stand facing each other with one slightly to the side. Place your elbow against the chest of the partner and without drawing your elbow back but by swinging and snapping up from your legs and through your hips explode your speed and force through your elbow and knock the partner backwards.

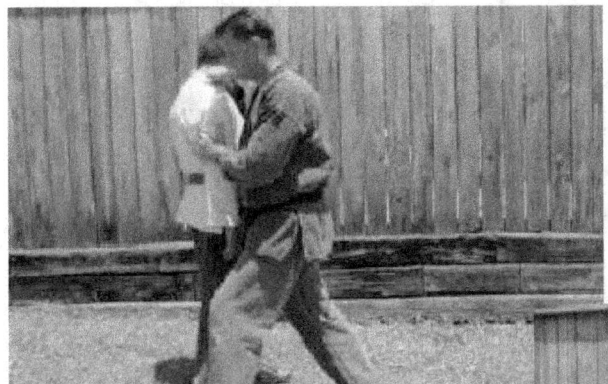

Elbow on the chest, ready position

Drawing the hips generating power in legs

Perform this exercise at least 15 times and continue daily till you have mastered this hip explosiveness.

Elbow Smashing: often in football the players will hit the opponent in the chest or block him using their elbows to swing up and hit the chest area. There will be a loud noise but usually not much damage. This is because you have very little strength that is available to use to raise your elbows straight up. Once your elbows are the level of the shoulder, they have almost no strength left in them. So to generate the most power from this blow, one should not lift his elbows any higher than the middle of the chest and use his legs and hips for the power generation to explode through the opponent. Simply snap through the legs and pop the hips up, keeping the elbows locked and arms unbendable and your force will be powerful and explosive.

No power in elbows or arms at this height. Notice partner can stop movement. Exploding through the hips and legs, locking arms for maximum power.

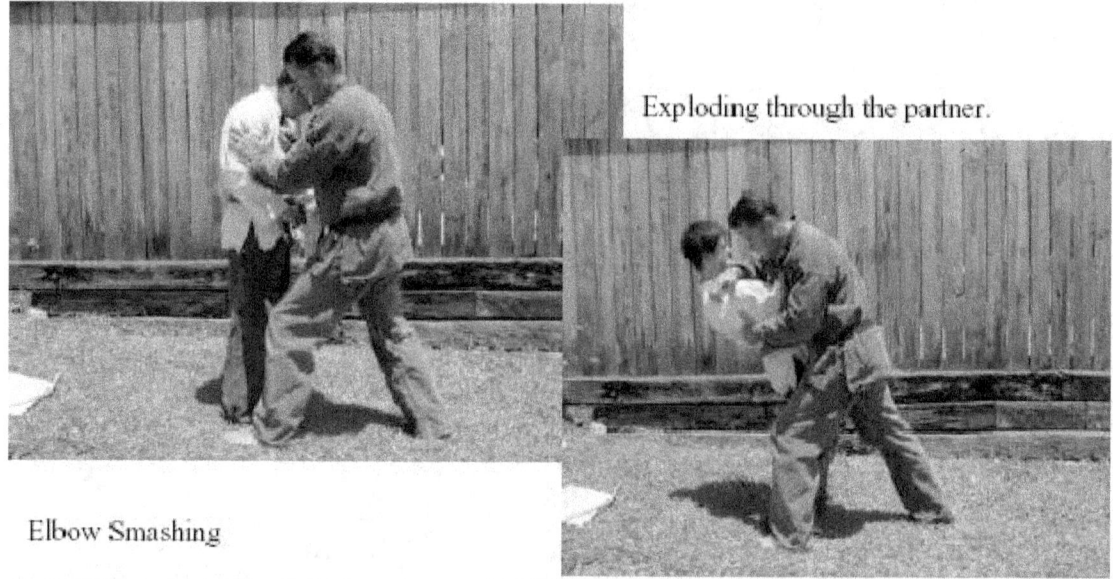

Exploding through the partner.

Elbow Smashing

The Elbow Smash: often just one elbow is used to hit the opponent, but this elbow loses most of its power if it is used simply as an arm and shoulder swing. If you will snap the hips and thrust the body weight into the strike, keeping the elbow near the body, you will be able to explode through the opponent and create much more power.

Improper elbow smash Hips are back, elbow and shoulder are forward away from body. So you generate no real power.

Proper elbow smashing. Hips thrusting forward, elbow close to body. A unified movement for maximum power.

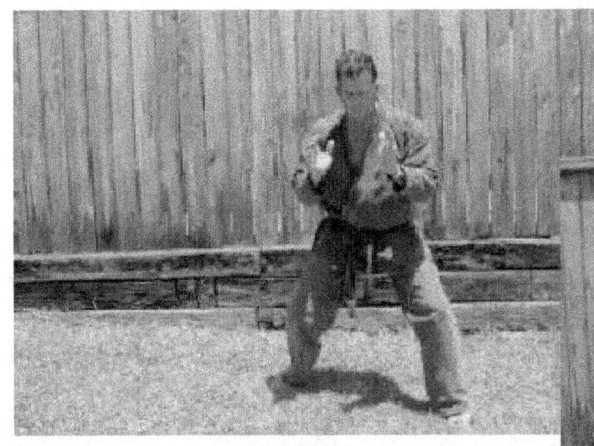

So to generate the most explosive power, begin to analyze your body positions when you are hitting someone or something and try to get as much of the hip movement and speed plus

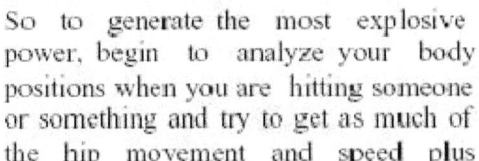

muscle into the blow as possible. Always exhale your air forcefully at the instant of impact. This allows for more muscle contraction and increased concentration with more power.

Steps in hip and body movement for power. Note the body moves as a unified group, snapping through the hips as the point of contact.

MartialArtsBusiness.com

"Where Martial Arts professionals go for answers 24 hours a day!"

V-001 • I-009
07/01

Register today for the Worldwide Martial Arts Business Expo! [see page 5 for details]

Cover Story

Interview with A Living Legend

PLUS...

Dealing With Problems
by Brian Tracy

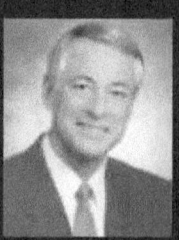

• INDUSTRY INSIDER • SELLNG • PERSONAL DEVELOPMENT • MARKETING • STAFF TRAINING •

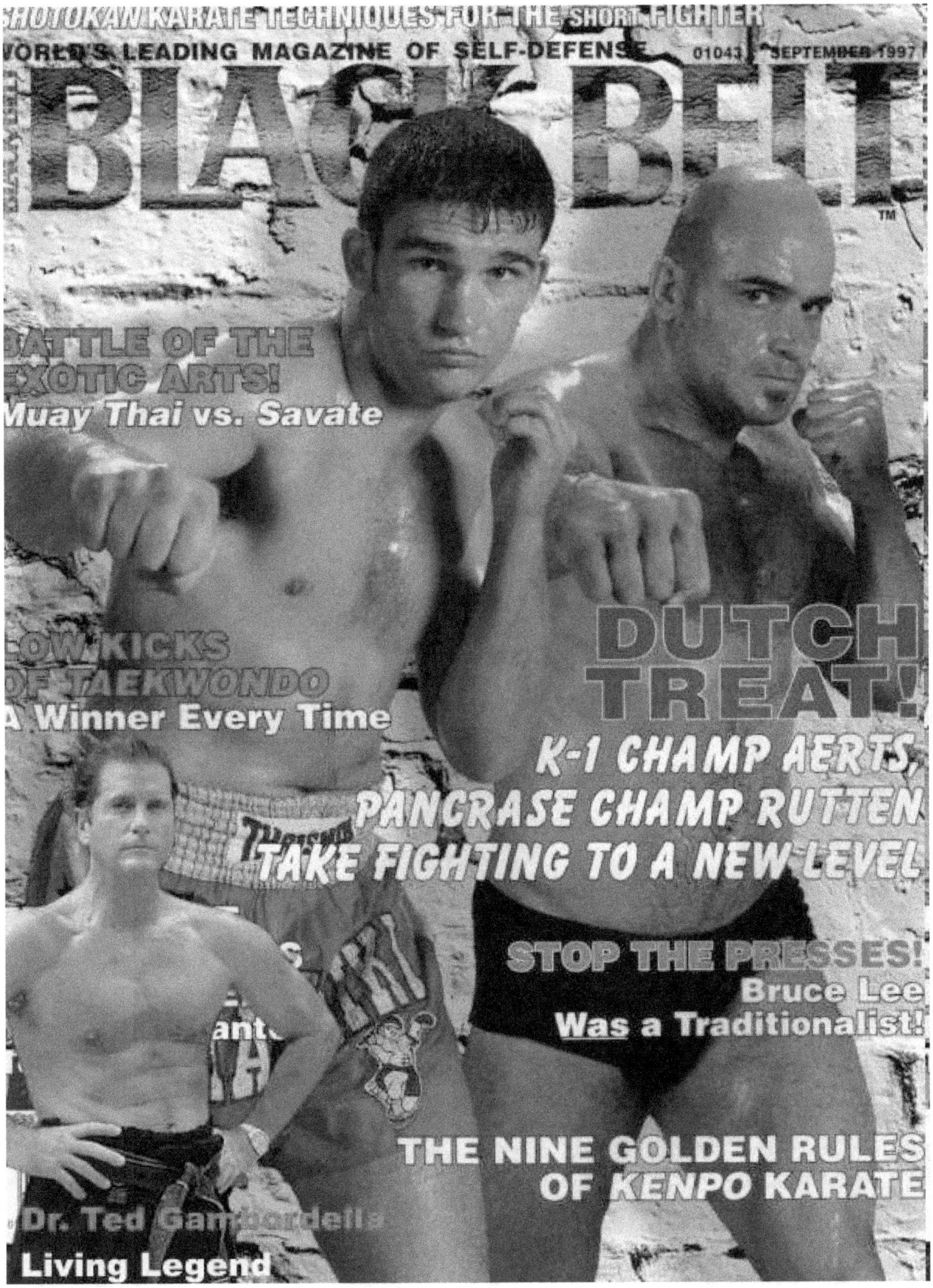

SHOTOKAN KARATE TECHNIQUES FOR THE SHORT FIGHTER

WORLD'S LEADING MAGAZINE OF SELF-DEFENSE   01043   SEPTEMBER 1997

BLACK BELT

BATTLE OF THE
EXOTIC ARTS!
Muay Thai vs. Savate

LOW KICKS
OF TAEKWONDO
A Winner Every Time

DUTCH TREAT!
K-1 CHAMP AERTS, PANCRASE CHAMP RUTTEN TAKE FIGHTING TO A NEW LEVEL

STOP THE PRESSES!
Bruce Lee
Was a Traditionalist!

THE NINE GOLDEN RULES
OF KENPO KARATE

Dr. Ted Gambordella
Living Legend

WIN! TRAINING EQUIPMENT, BOOKS AND VIDEOS!

INSIDE
KARATE

THE **DEADLY**
ELBOW OF MUAY THAI

WOMEN
CAN FIGHT!

MASTER
TATSU

Jiu Jitsu Expert
Dr. Ted Gambordella

INSIDE WIN

Jackie Chan's *The Myth !*

See Page 73

KUNG-FU

Down 'N Dirty
STREET COMBAT!

WHITE EYEBROW'S
SECRET STEPS!

MASTER JKD'S
HIGH-RISK
SPARRING!

SPECIAL REPORT!
MEXICO:
Kung-Fu's Next Hotbed?

IKF HALL HONORS
Grandmaster Ted Gambordella

FEBRUARY
U.S. $4.9

insidekung-fu.com

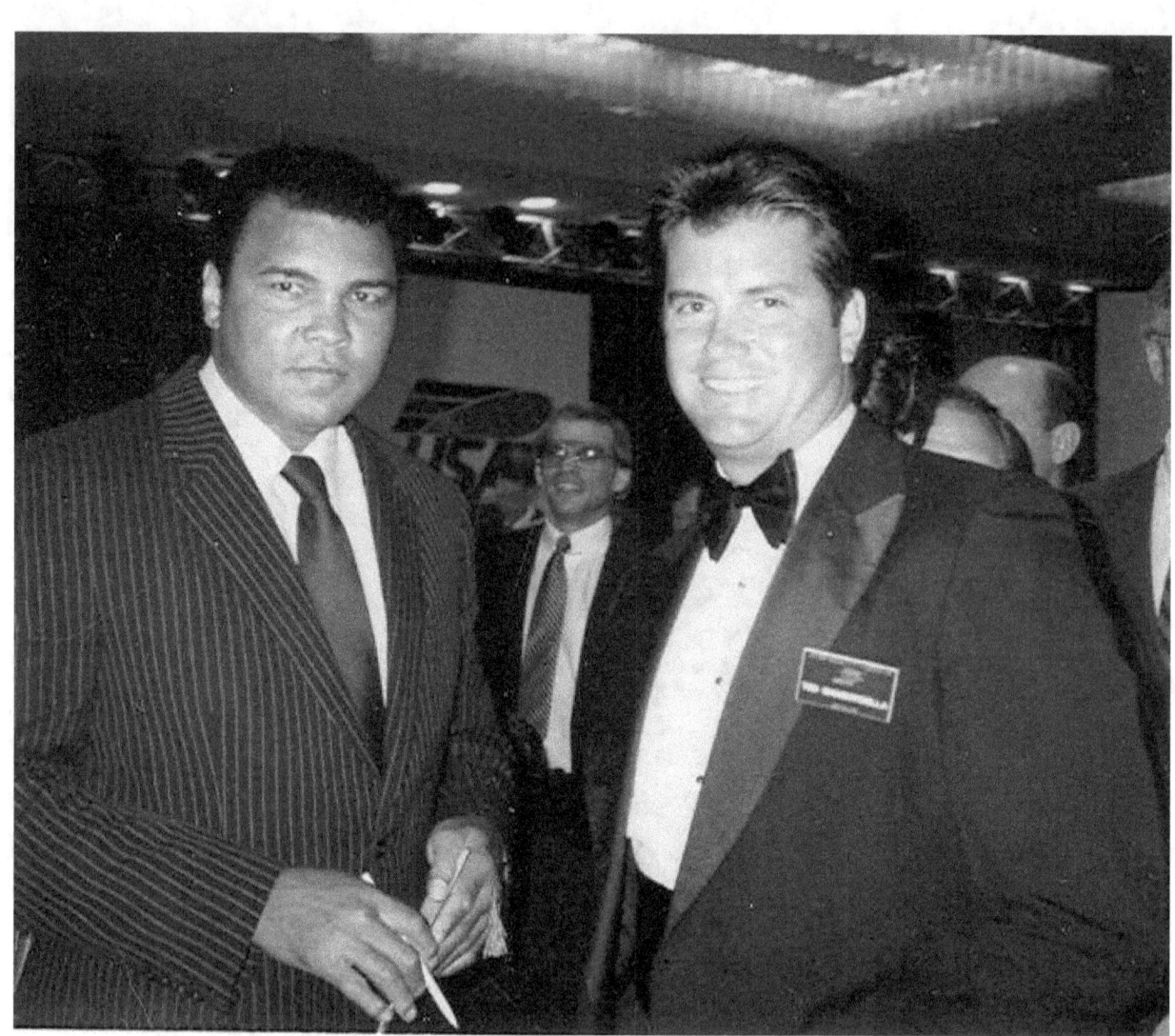

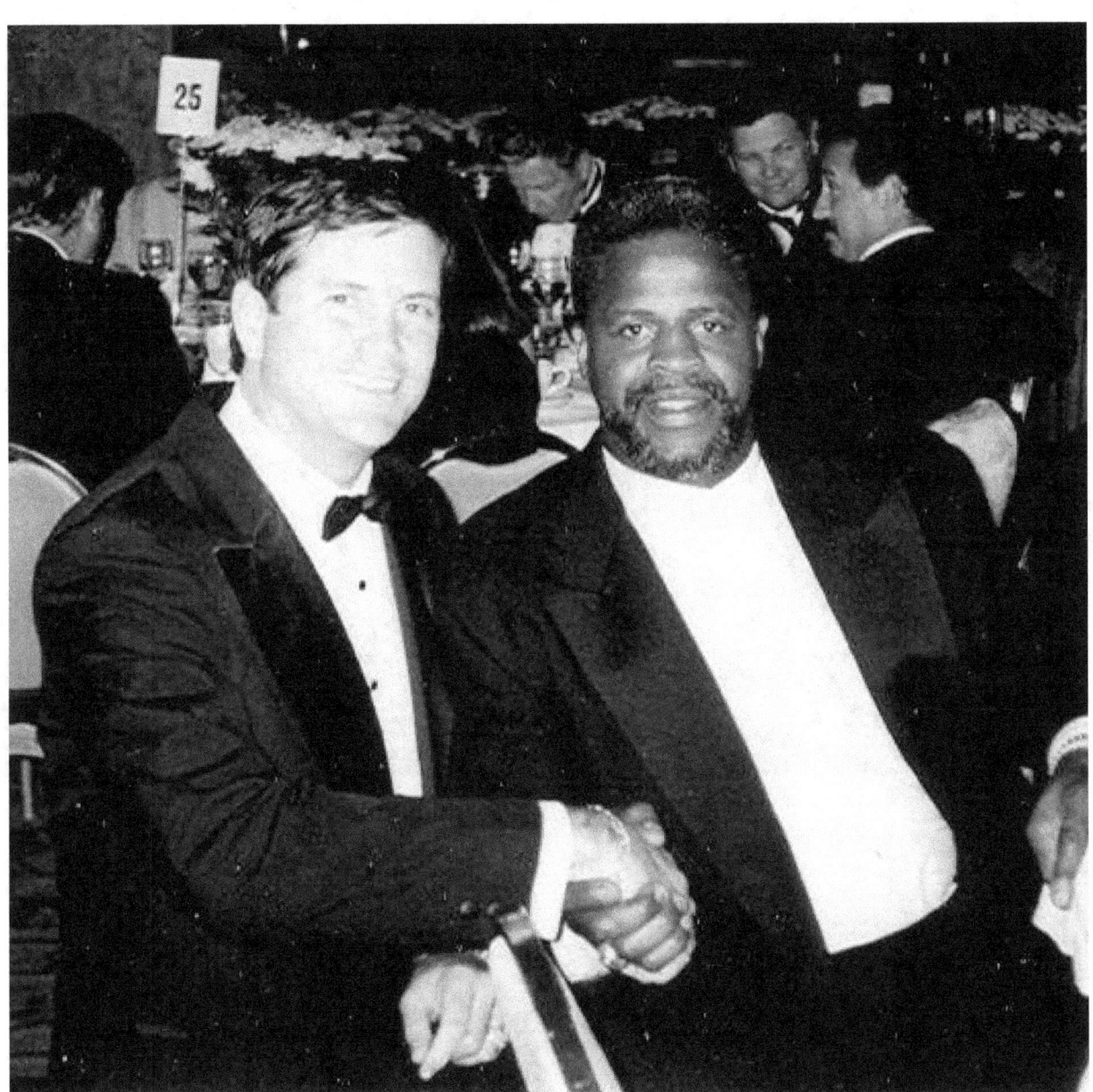

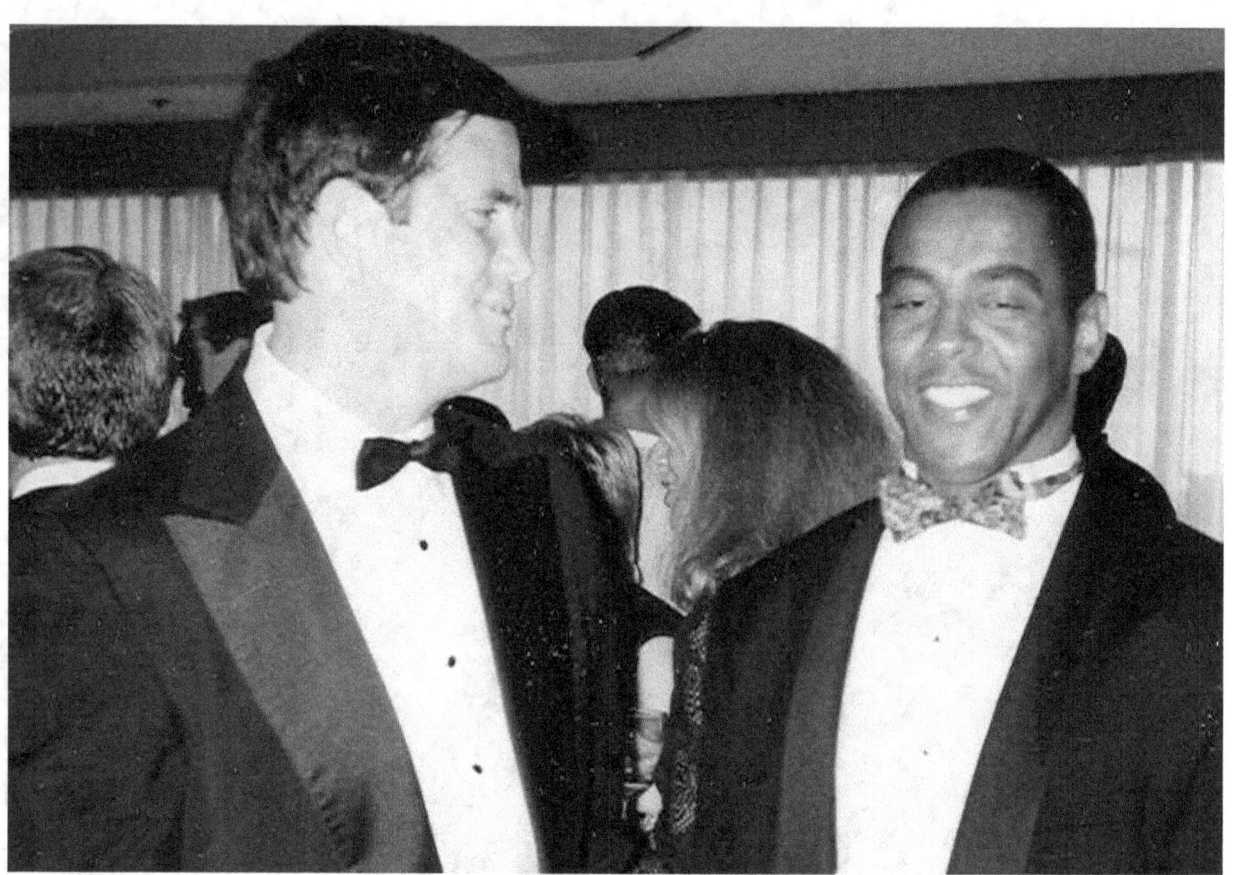

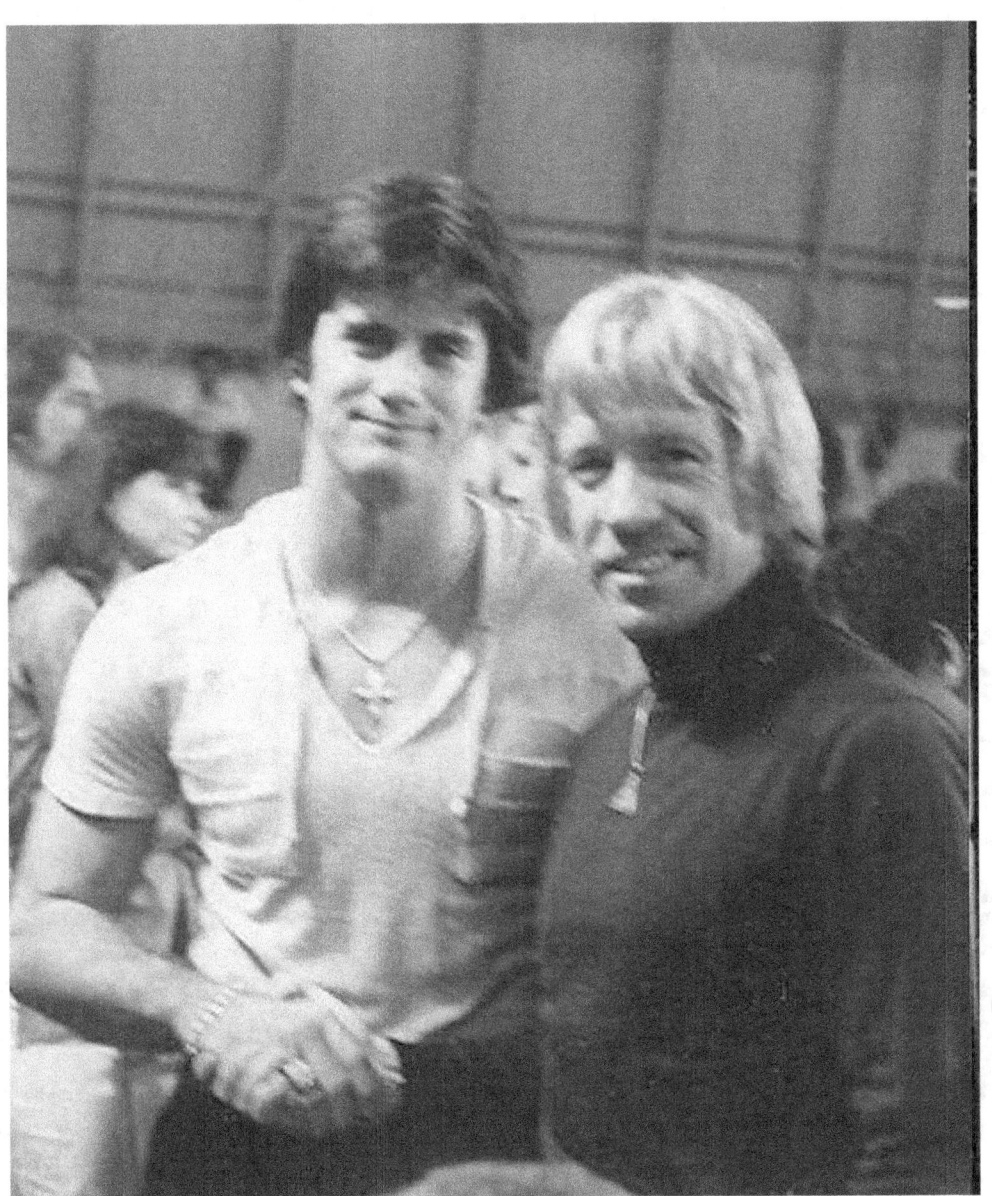

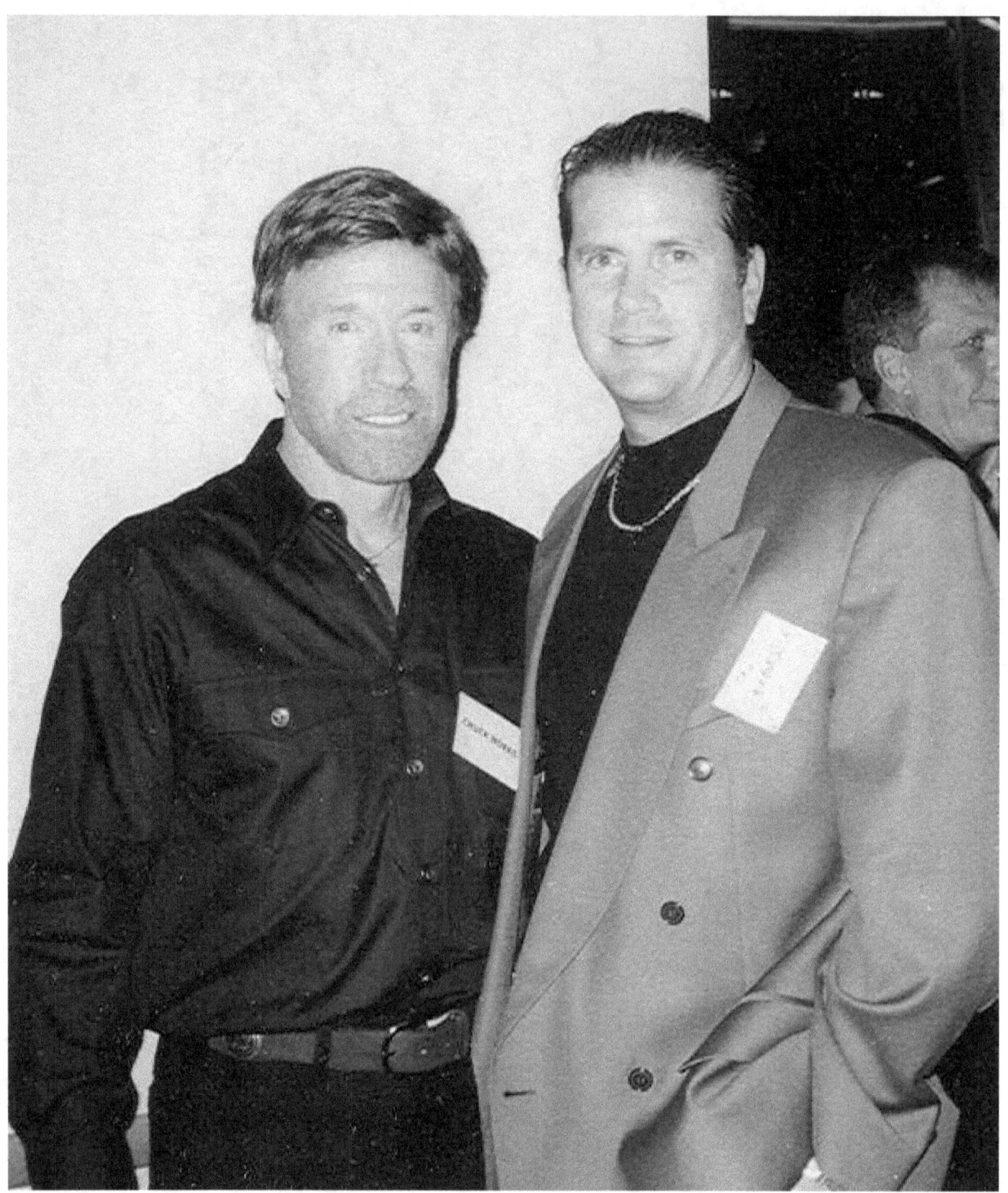

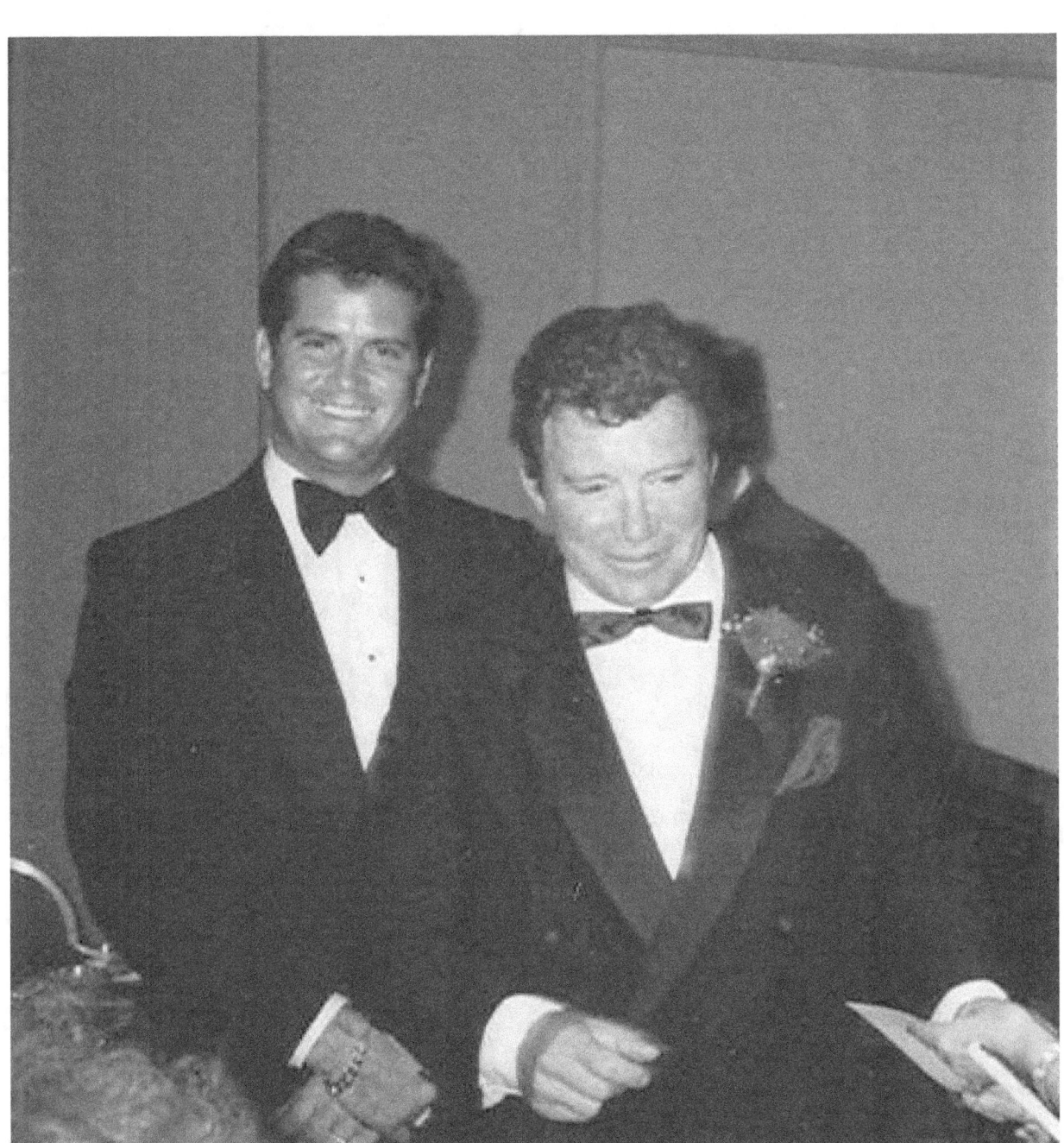

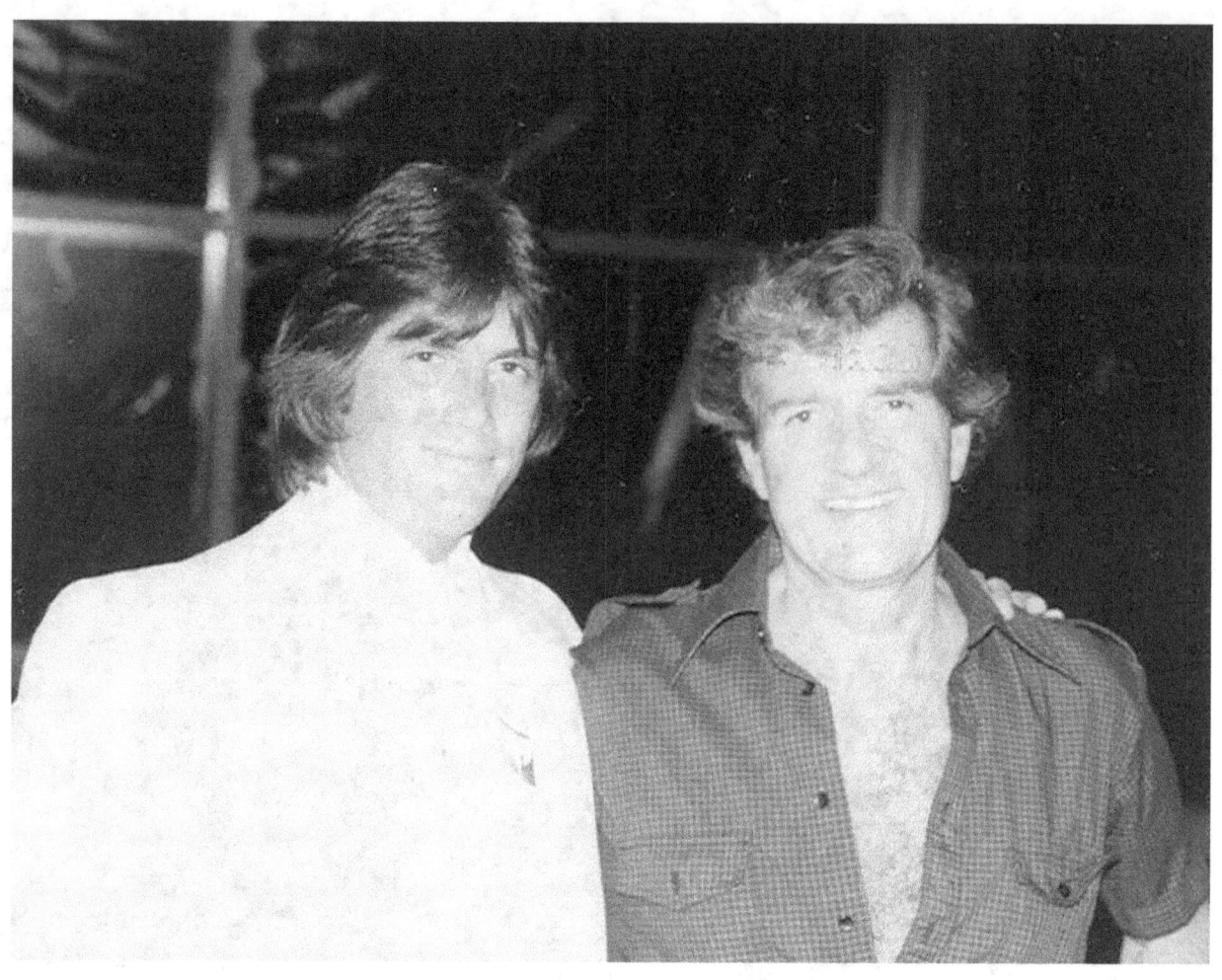

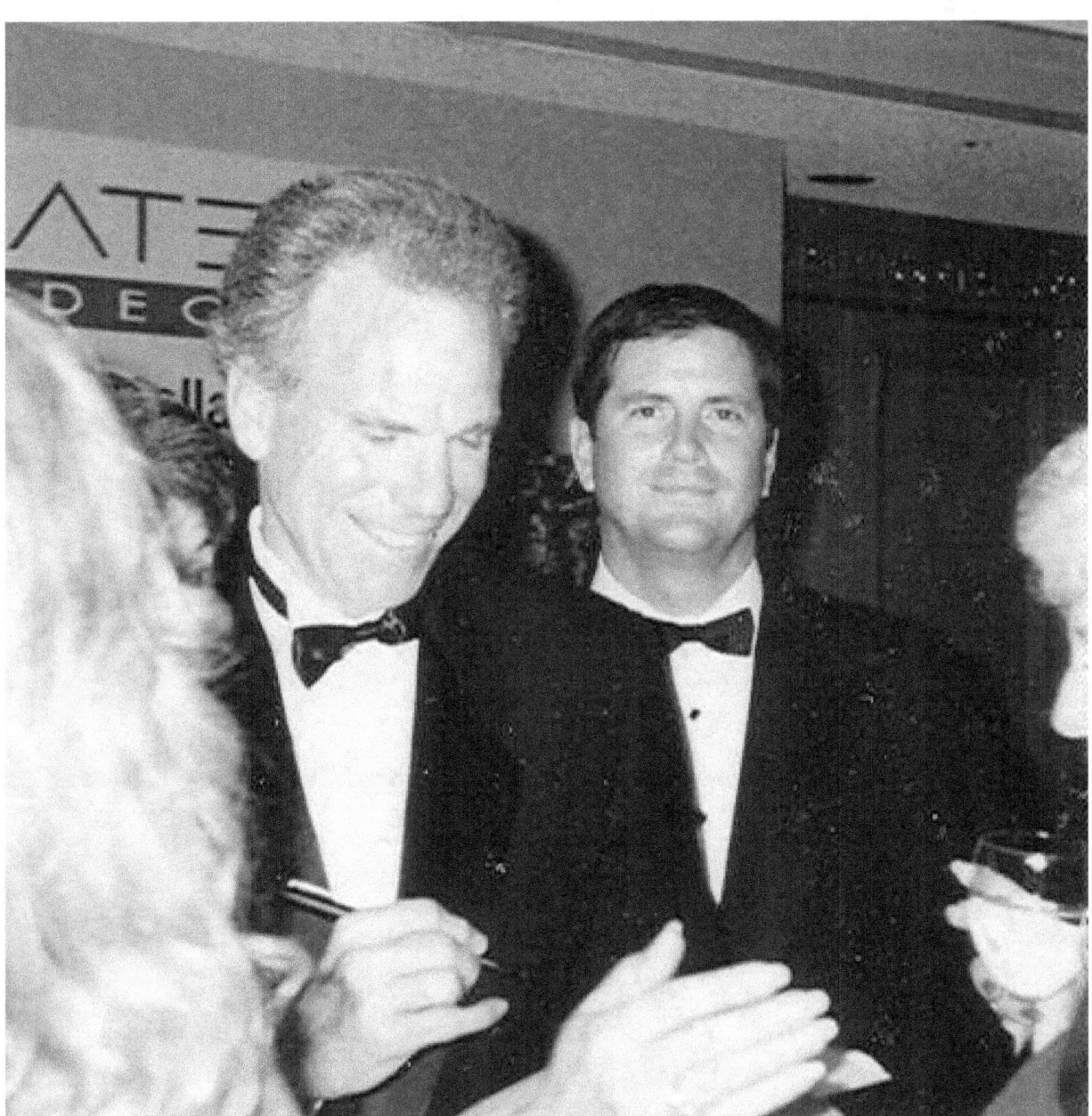

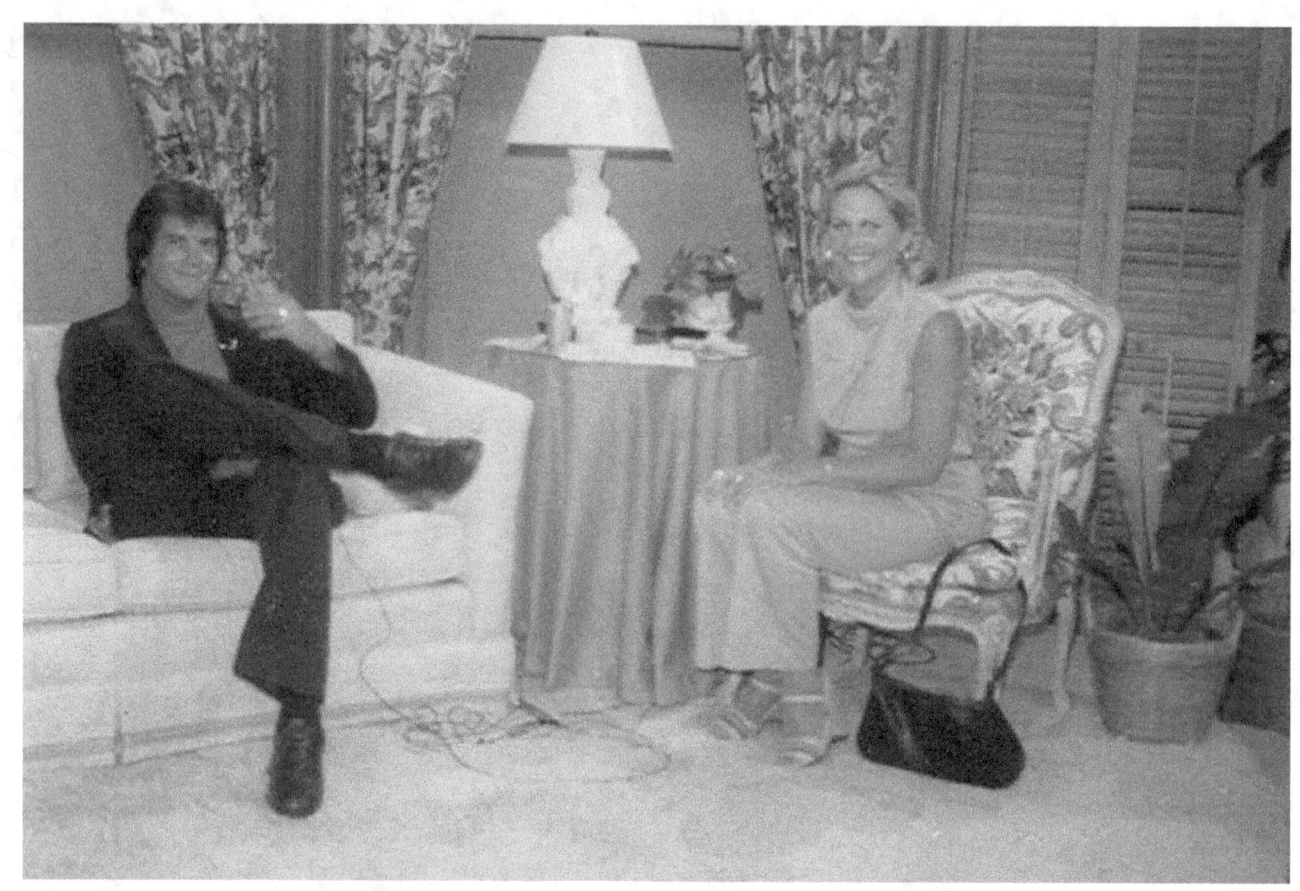

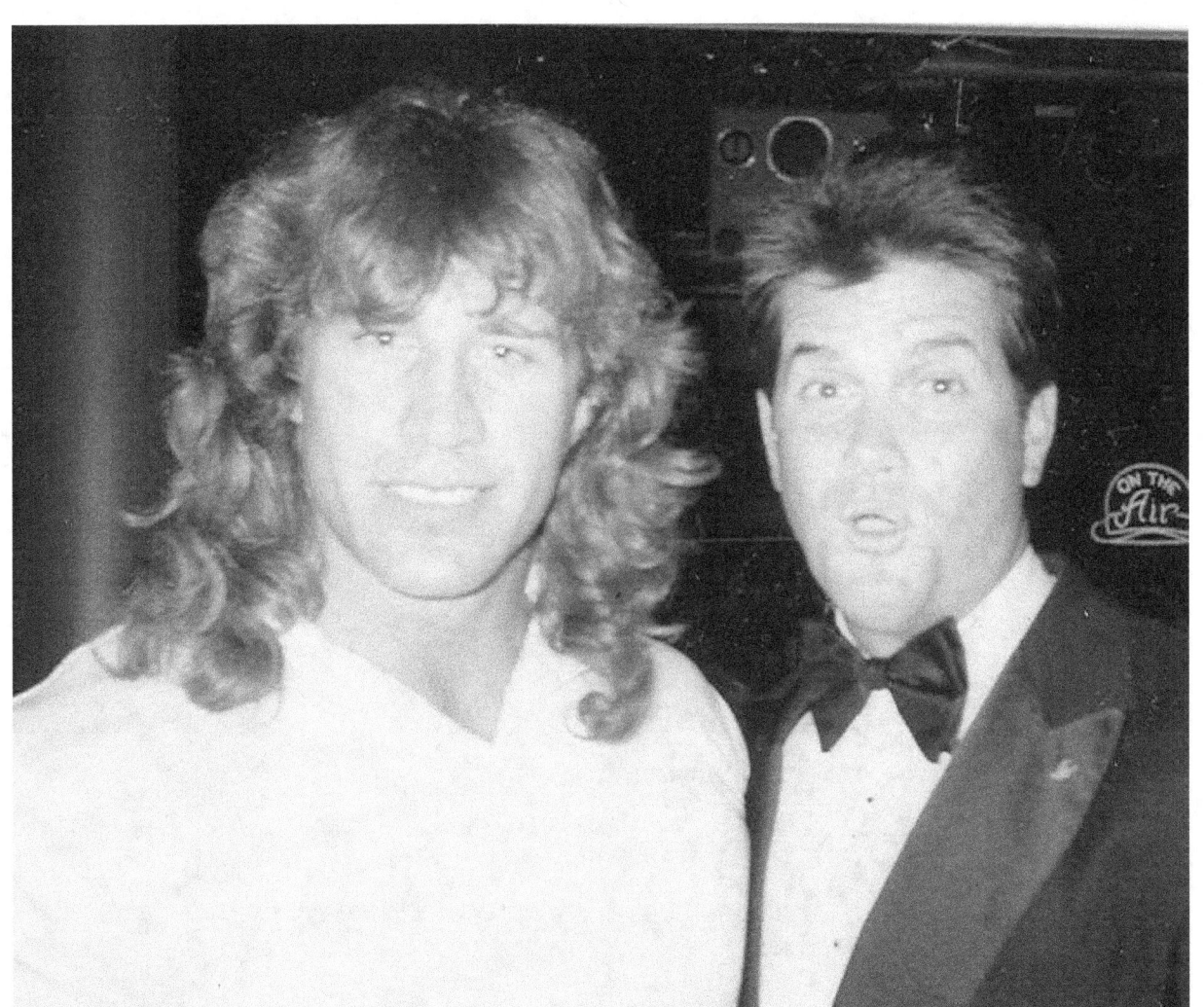

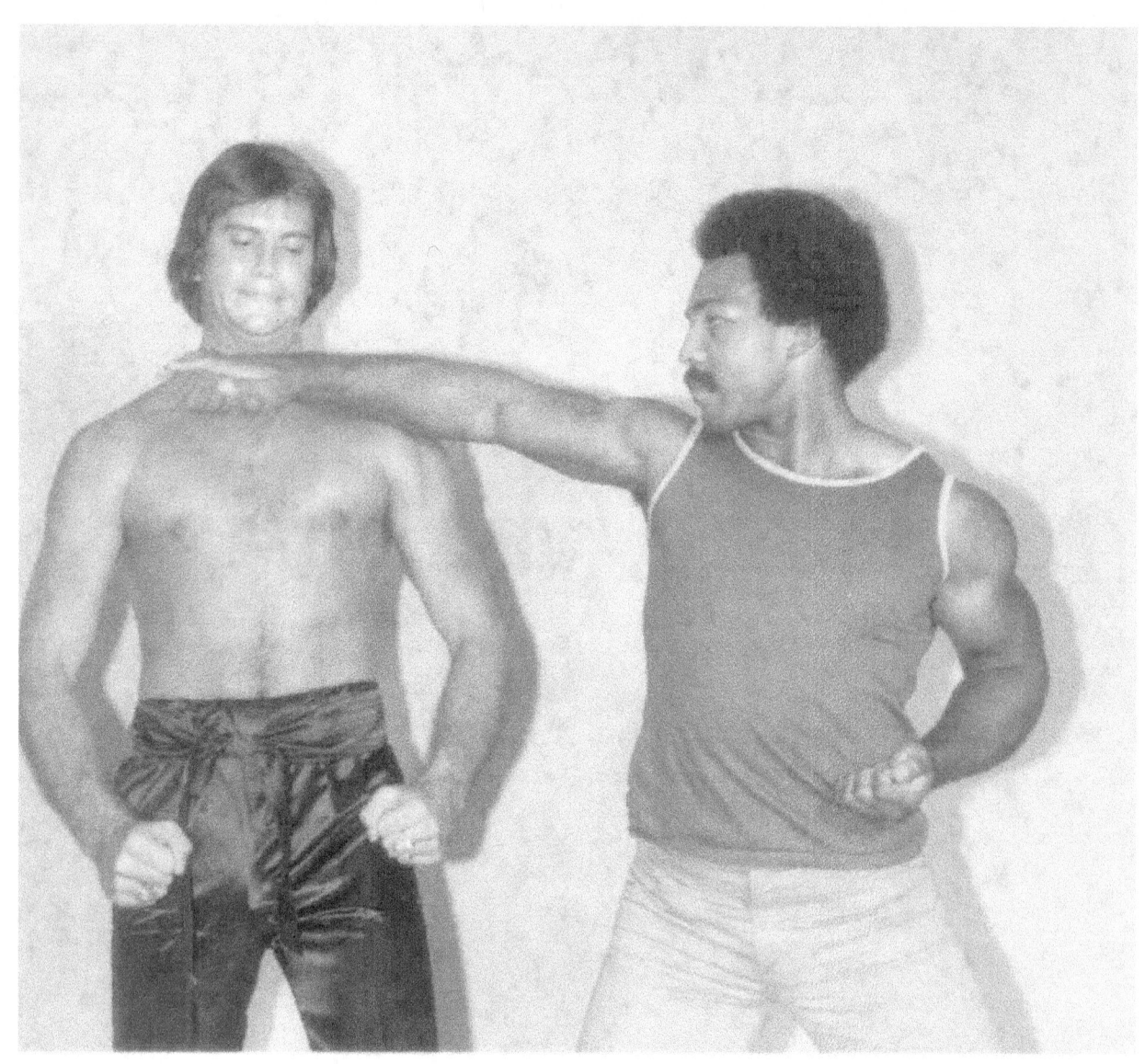

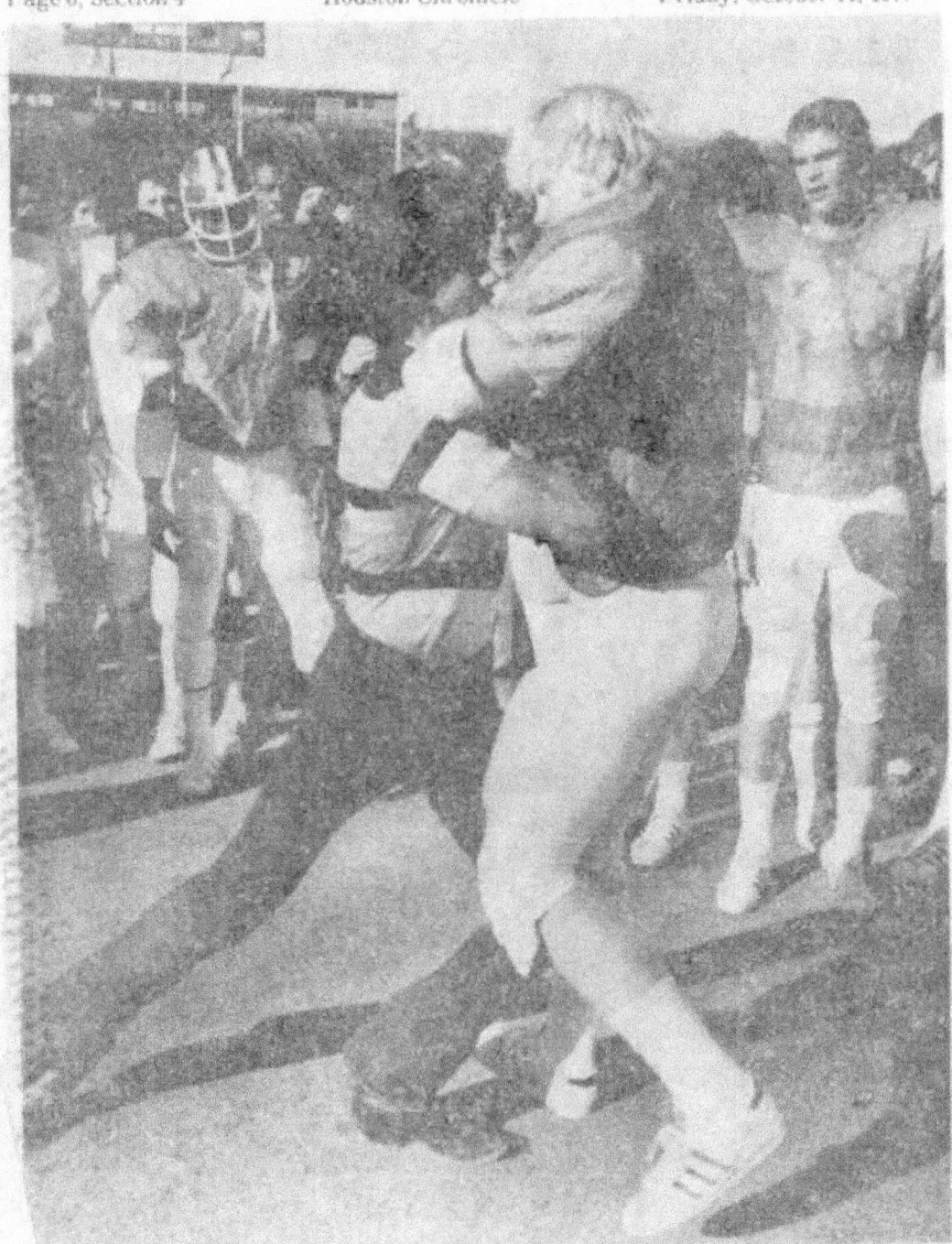

Photo by Mike Robinson, Chronicle Staff

Grrrrrrrrrr

...do expert Ted Gambordella
...monstrates a block on Rice
...tball player Joey Bevill.

Gammbordella explained balance points to the Owls Thursday at Rice Stadium.

he really wowed the kids. They were very happy with him. He took our biggest player, 6-foot-10, 250 pounds, and had him hit him in the ribs as hard as he could. He wore the basketball player out, and his hand was all bloody. But Gambordella didn't even budge. There was hardly a mark.

"I get a million guys in here with a gimmick, with everything from machines to pills. Guys who say they'll make the players jump over the moon or run through the Berlin Wall. But I do not think he is a quack. I think his thesis is good.

"His theory is not a new one, just his way of presenting it. His greatest contribution is his mental imagery theory." Brown's team led the Southeastern Conference in rebounding last year, and said he'd

the players what they can do when they get hit.

Winston Duke, Richardson High's football coach, agrees.

"If we didn't believe in him, we wouldn't have brought him in," Duke said. "I'll say this, he gave the kids enough confidence to take a lick, and not come off the field every time they got hit. He did a good job with everything he did, and he probably helped most of our kids. We didn't have any major injuries at all this year."

Rice, isn't sure whether he'll bring Gambordella to Cincinnati, although the Bengals would seem to need a lot of help. "I think there's a lot to this," Rice said.

Now if Gambordella can just find that publisher.

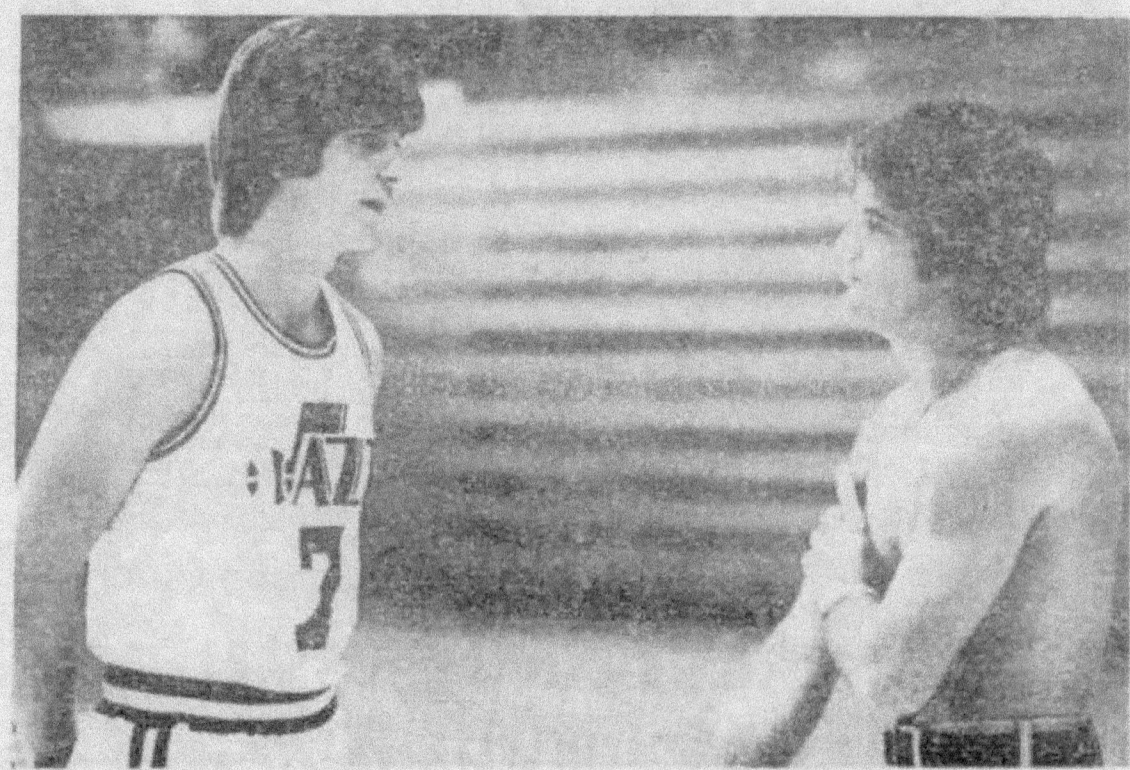

Jazz players couldn't touch their toes — not even Pete Maravich

FRII

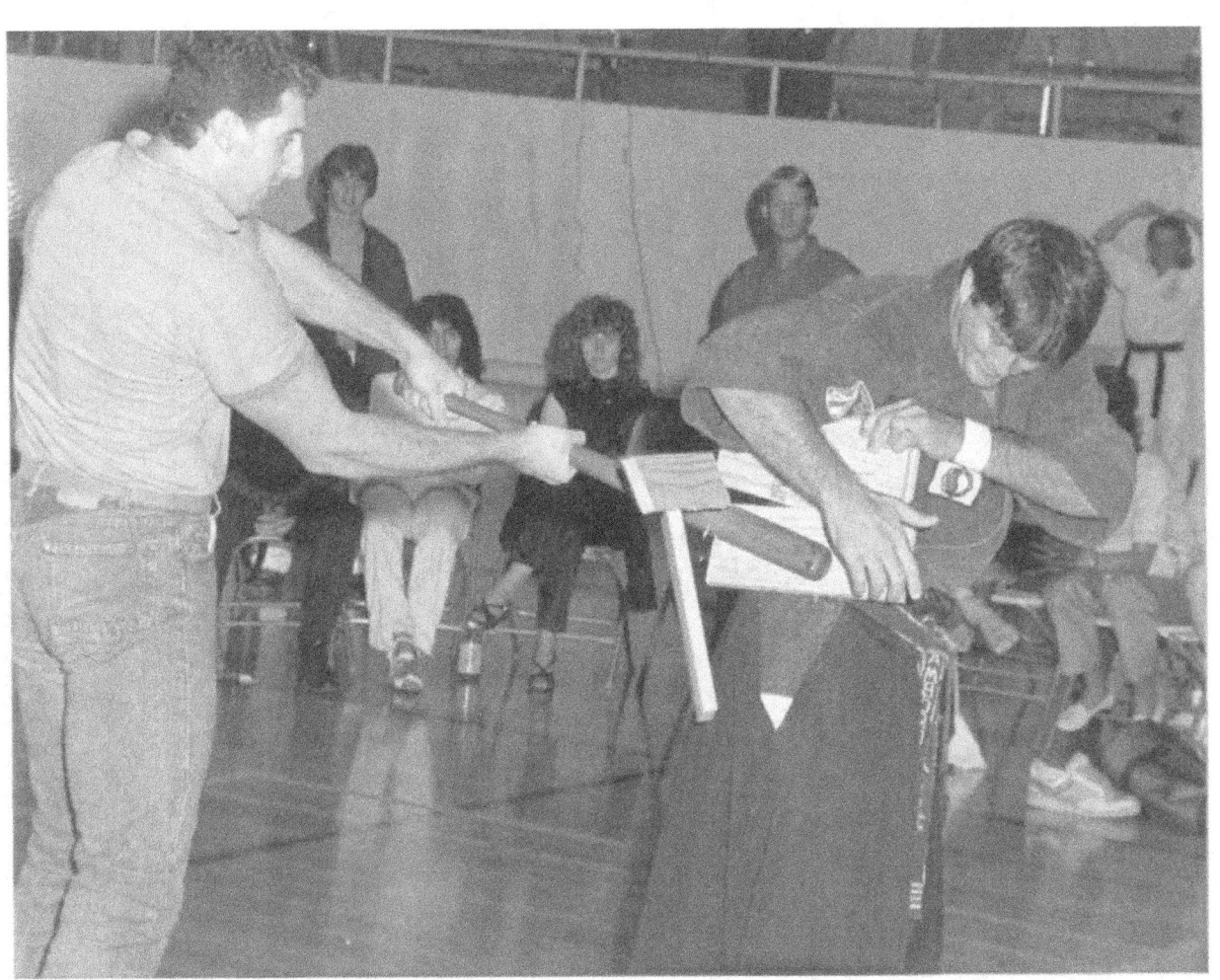

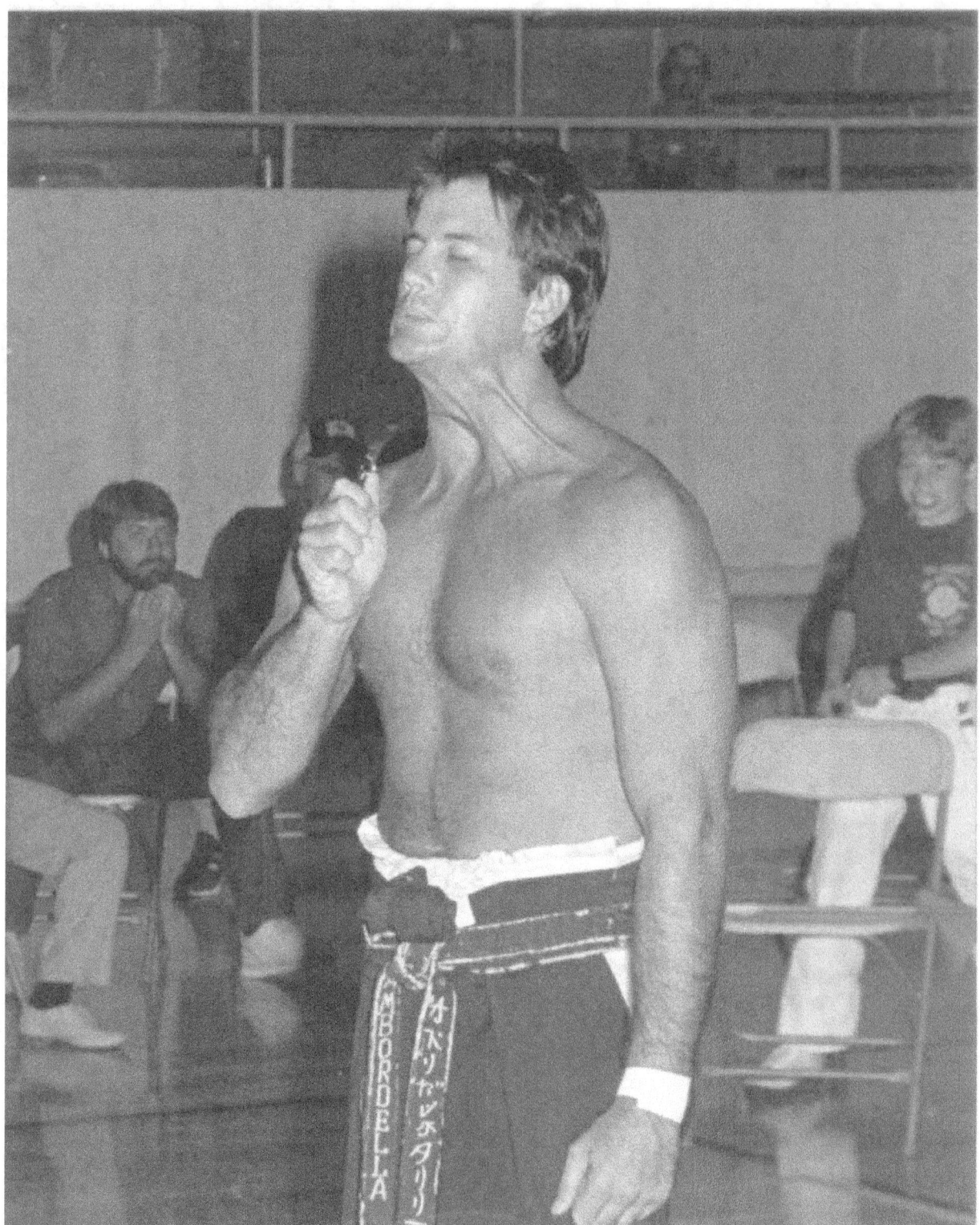

L.S.U. COLLEGIATE KARATE CHAMPIONSH

SUNDAY, NOVEMBER 16, 1975

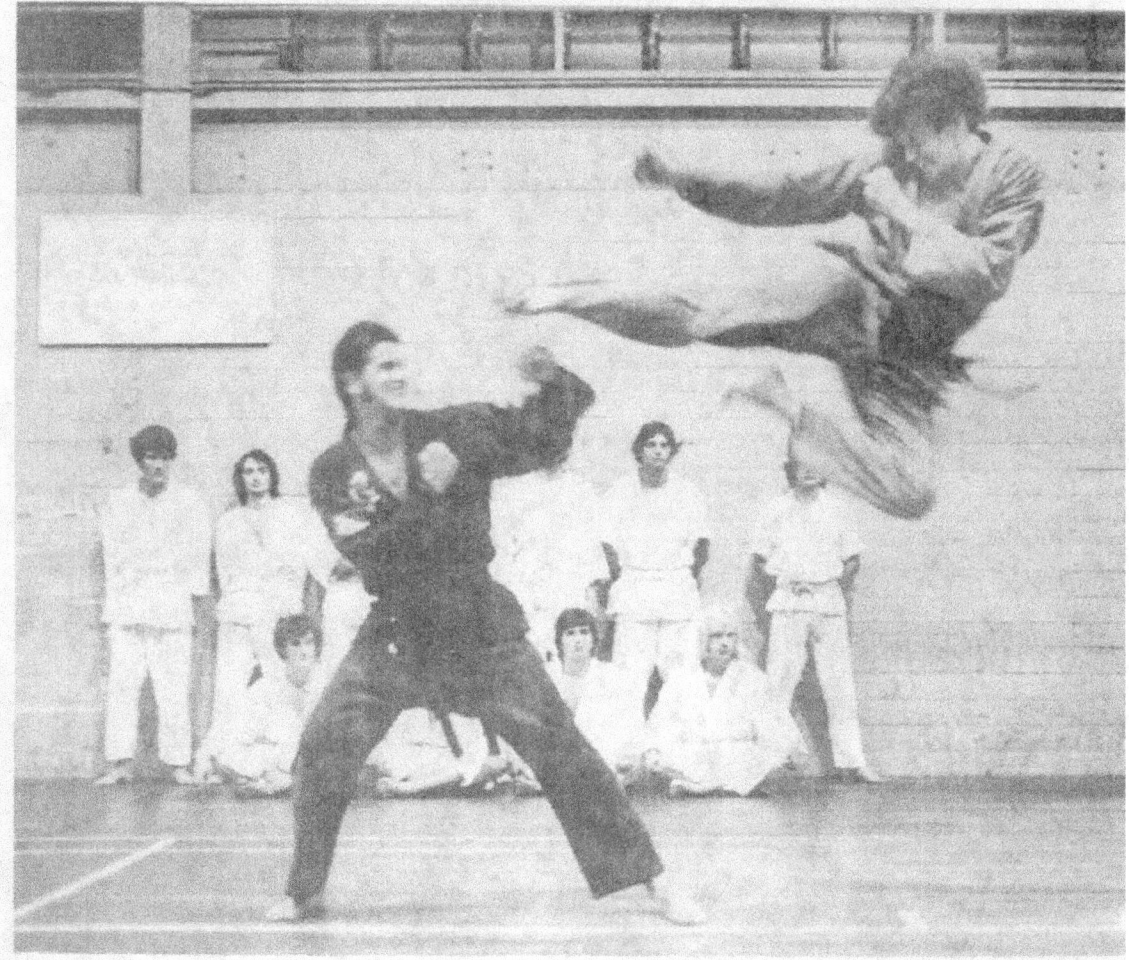

GYM ARMORY

tastic Demonstrations   Registration 8:00—9:

d vs. pain) training

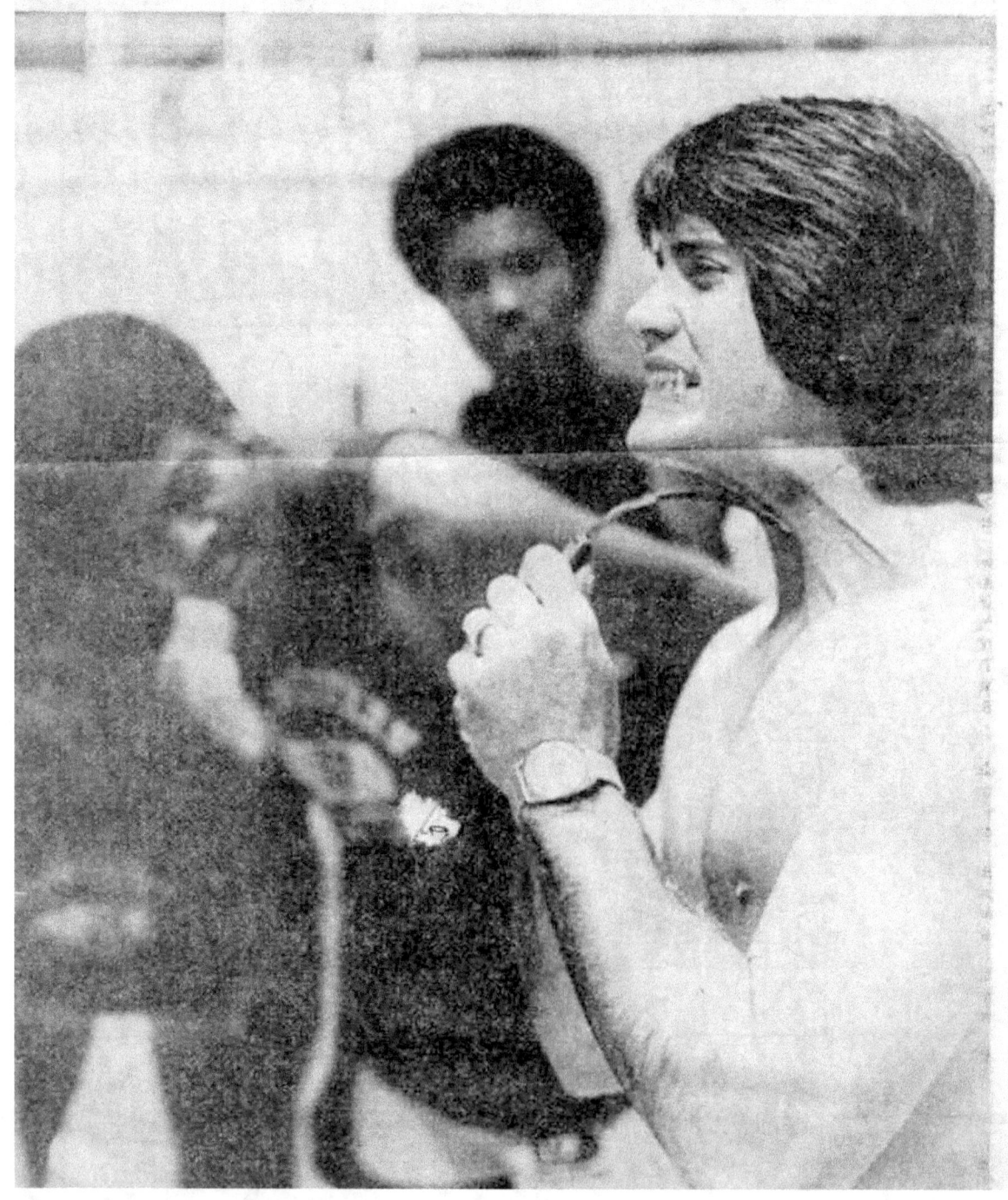

Jiu-Jitsu

Players learn mind control

By Doug Brown

If the Midwestern basketball players look like they are in another world when they take the court this year it is due to the jiu-jitsu technique of mind control being taught to the squad by Ted Gambordella.

Gambordella, manager and part-owner of a local spa, is teaching the Midwestern squad the techniques and control of the mind through jiu-jitsu.

"It teaches you breath and muscle control and dicipline of the mind," Gambordella said.

Midwestern basketball coach Gerald Stockton hopes the method will help the players become more aware of the game's mental attitude and prevent nagging injuries from hampering the player's performances.

With the jiu-jitsu mind control an individual can endure pain enough to concentrate on his performance in a game.

"Jui-jitsu can give a person greater endurance, flexibility and enables the basketball player to withstand the contact under the basket," Gambordella said.

An eight-year veteran of the martial arts, Gambordella has earned five Black Belts, three in jui-jitsu and one each in karate and kempo.

Gambordella has taught self-defense courses in hospitals, high schools, colleges and various organizations.

After tutoring the Midwestern players, Gambordella plans to teach self-defense courses in the dorms and sororities.

"A person can learn to withstand punches to any part of the body, including the throat and ribs, in three months," Gambordella said.

The average person can become more flexible, more fearless and prevent pain in any part of the body, Gambordella said.

Gambordella attended the karate olympics and taught athletes the jiu-jitsu form of mind control.

Among the demonstrations he performs are various ways to withstand a punch to the ribs and throat and using razor sharp knives to demonstrate the strength of the neck muscles.

In 1974-75, Gambordella coached the Louisiana State University karate team to the Southern Collegiate Karate championship.

"I think that we could start a Midwestern karate team that could compete on the collegiate level," Gambordella said.

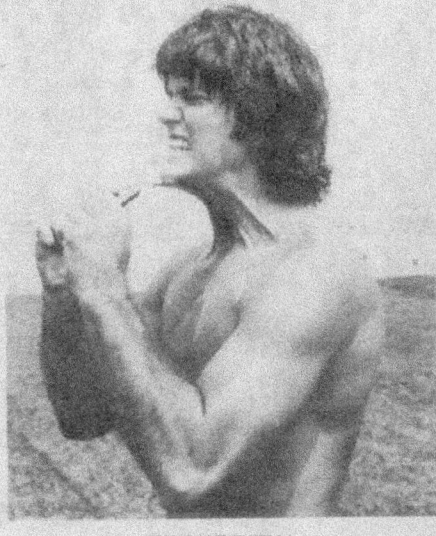

TED GAMBORDELLA
...Knives applied to the neck show strength of muscles.

MSU women drop games

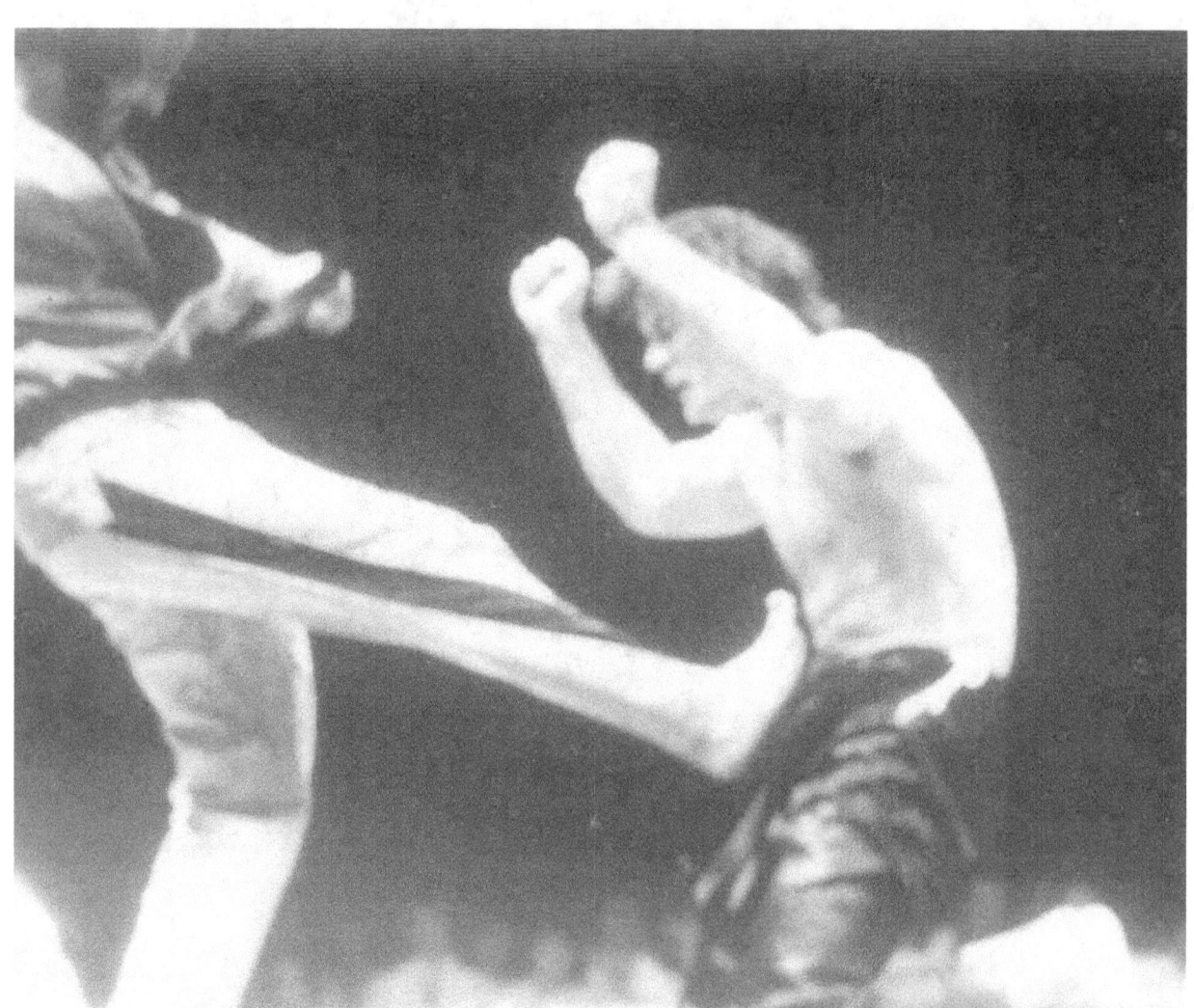

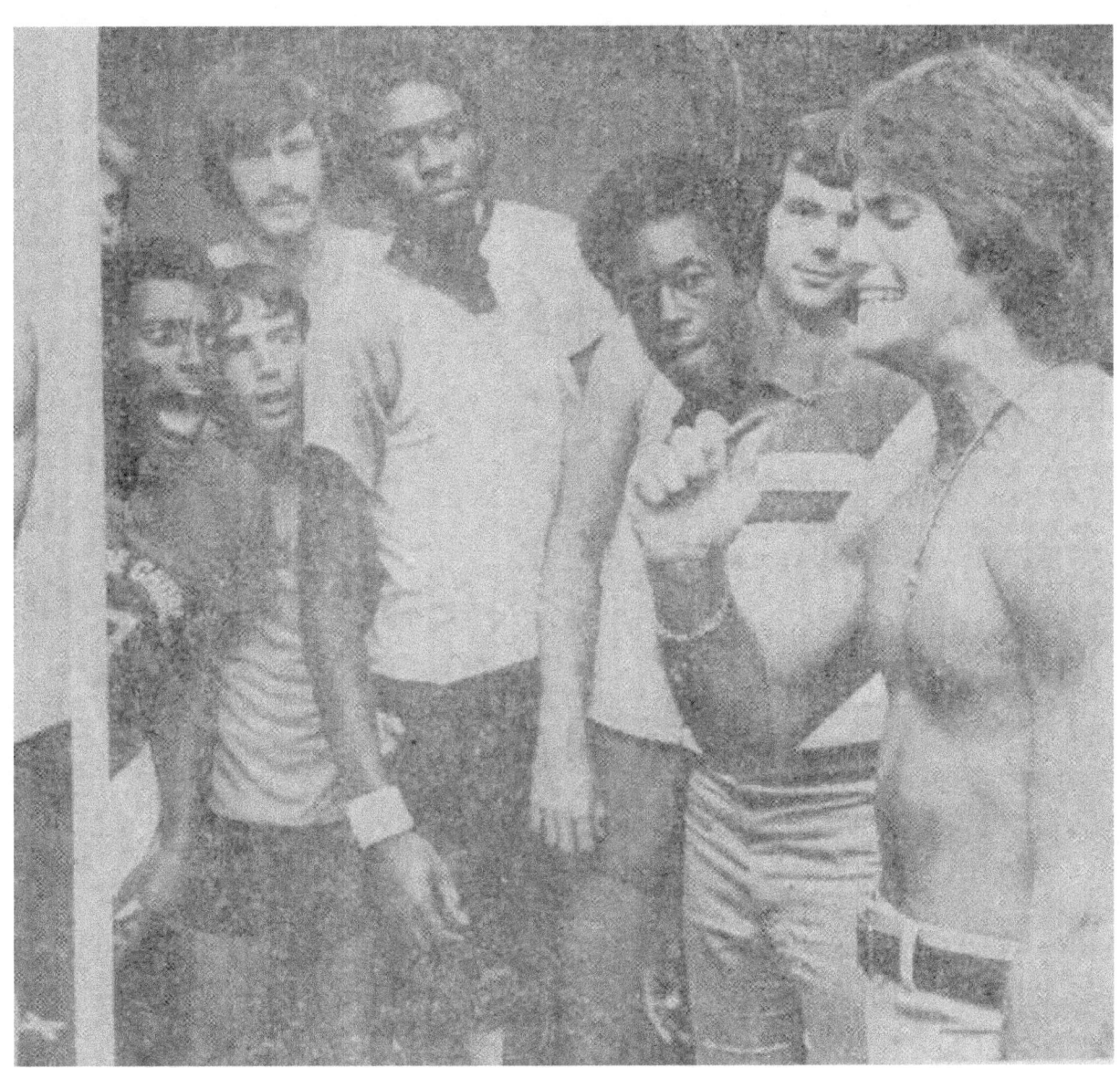

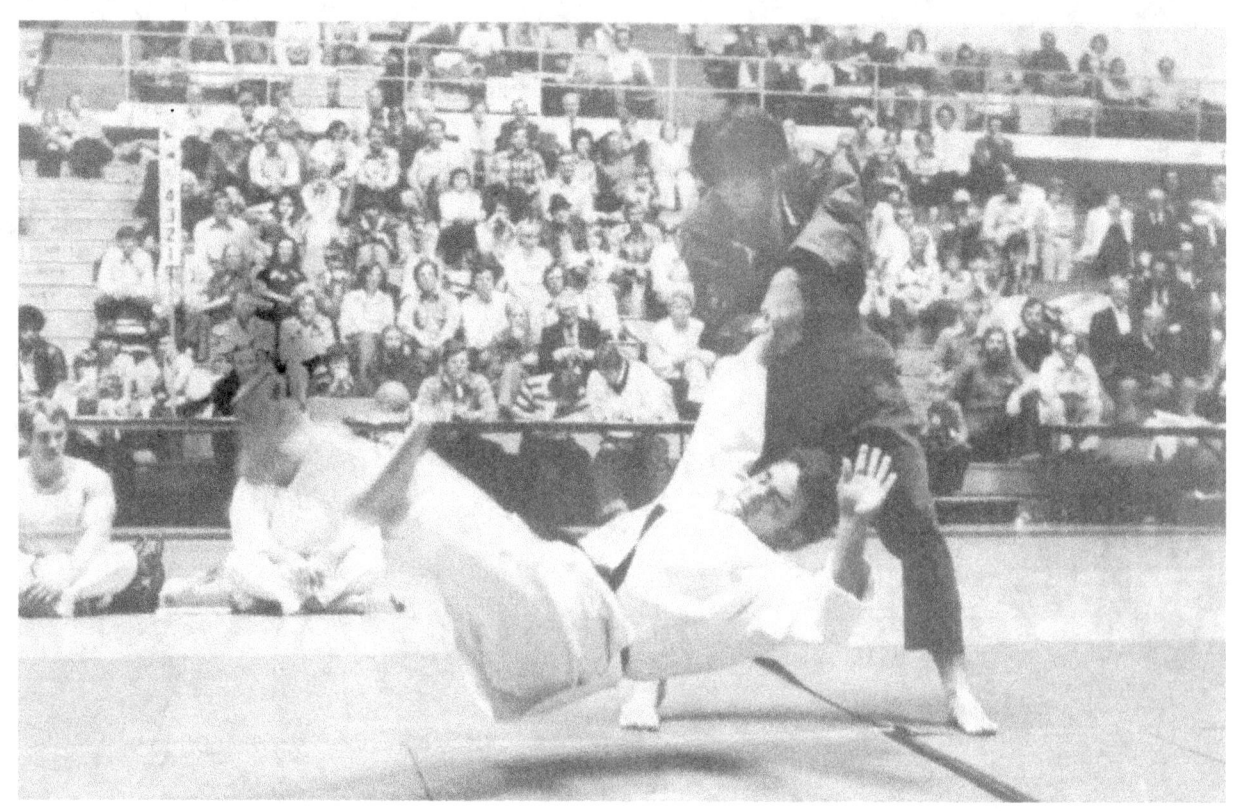

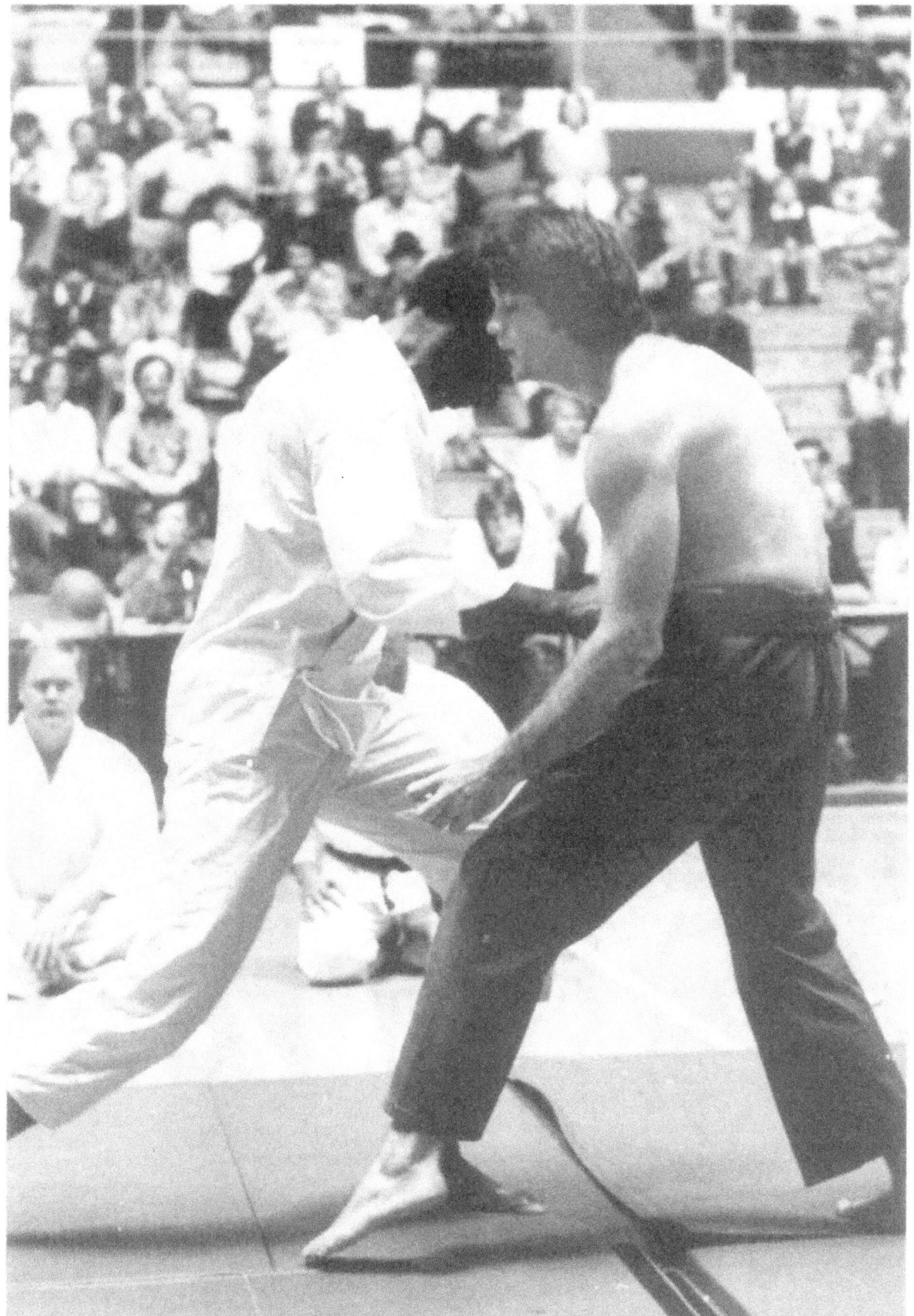

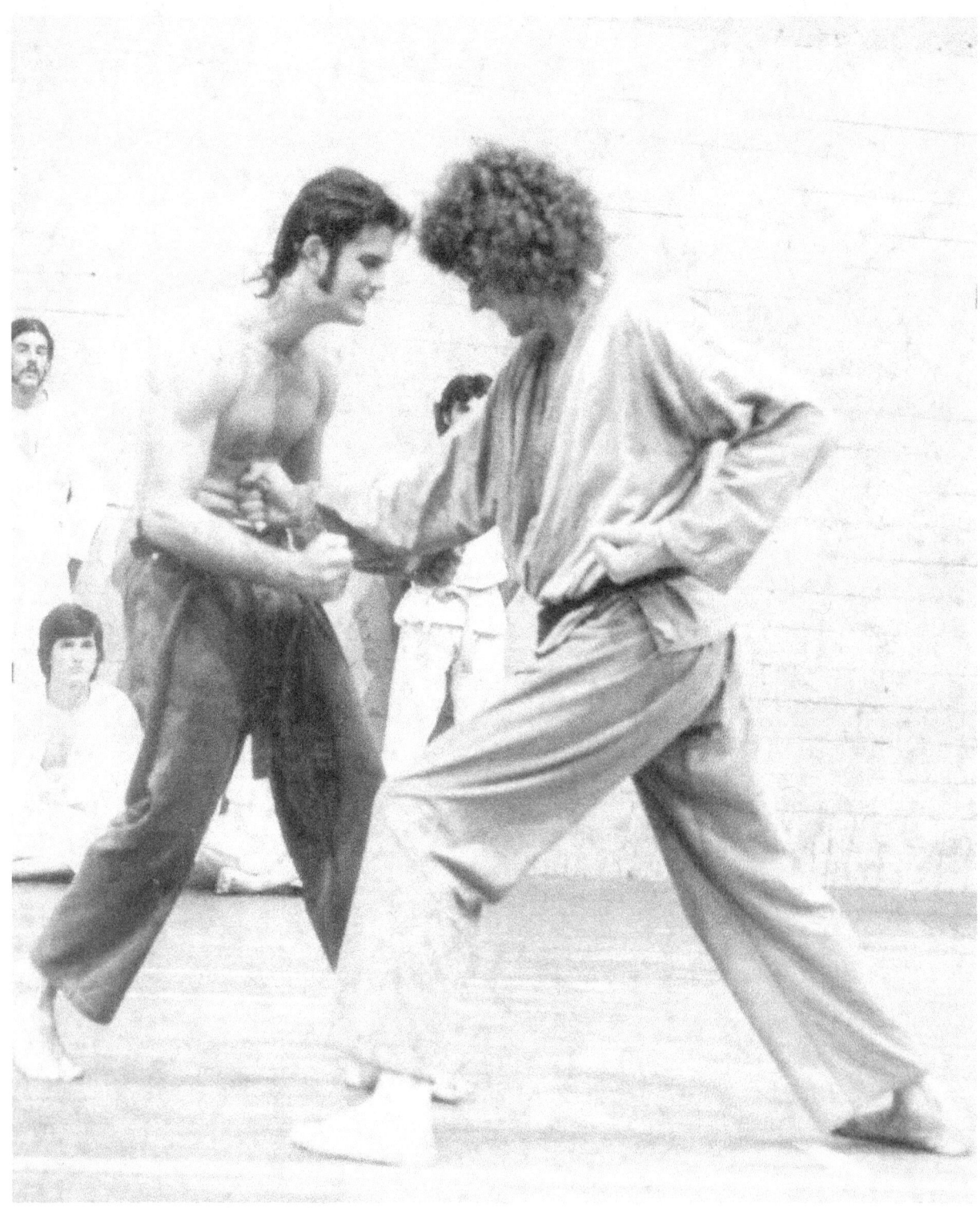

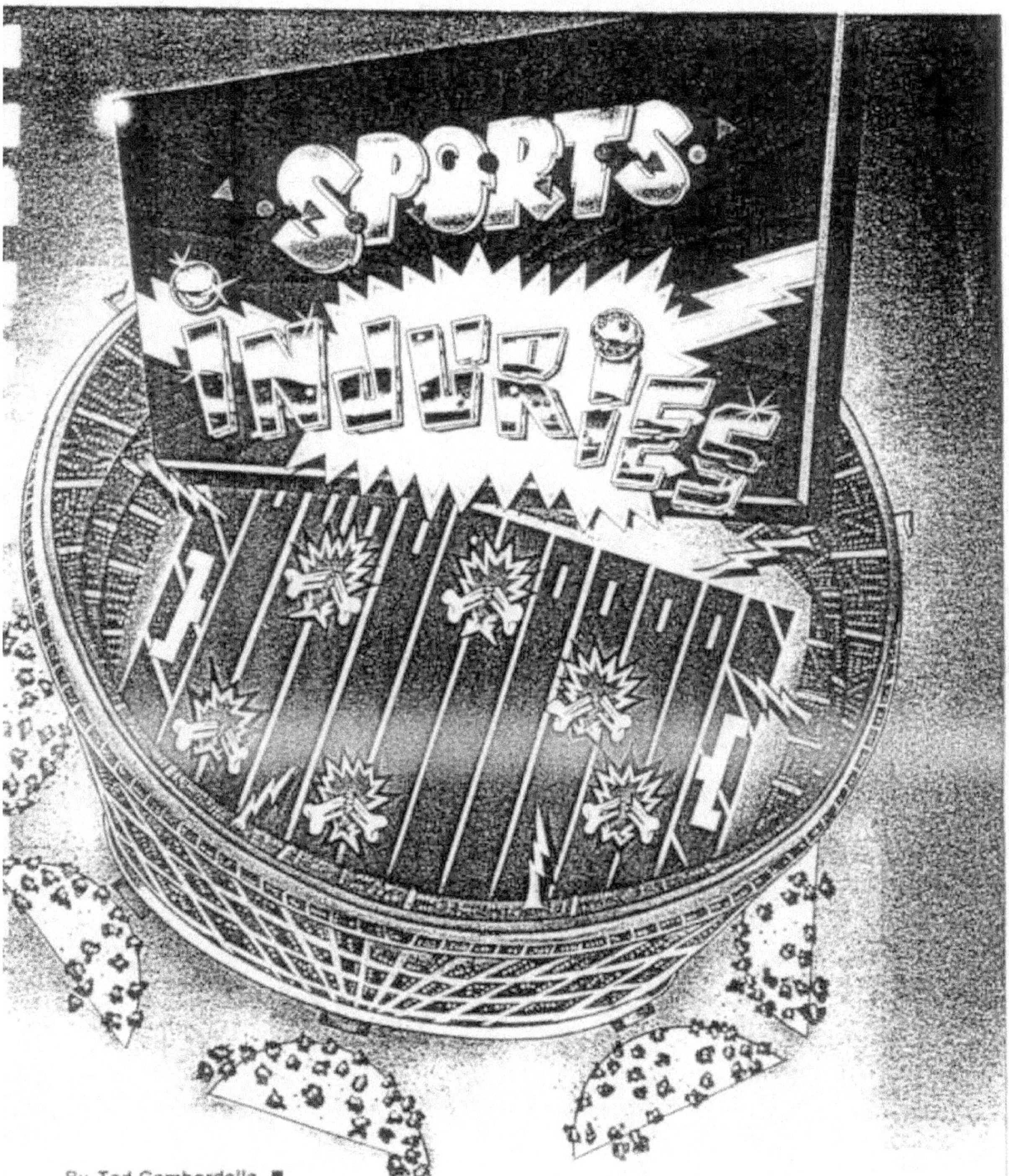

By Ted Gambordella

Sports injuries plague thousands of people each year. Professional athlete just a weekend warrior, you face possible serious injury. But by practicing a few simple and easy-to-learn techniques, you can sharply reduce your chances of sports injury.

Americans are sports crazy —everyone loves sports. And many people think that part of the game is the risk of injury, but that everything that can be done to prevent needless injuries is being done. A few injuries per game can be expected, and although we really don't like to see them happen, it just wouldn't be the same if no one got hurt. In fact, violence is one of the main drawing cards in professional sports.

But not everyone realizes just how violent sports really are, or how many Americans have died during athletic competition. The problem hasn't been completely ignored, and has, at times, attracted the attention of the U.S. government. In fact, in 1905, 18 young men died playing college football alone; which prompted Theodore Roosevelt to issue a Presidential decree that football should "square itself away" or become outlawed. More recent statistics show the following: in 1968 there were 31

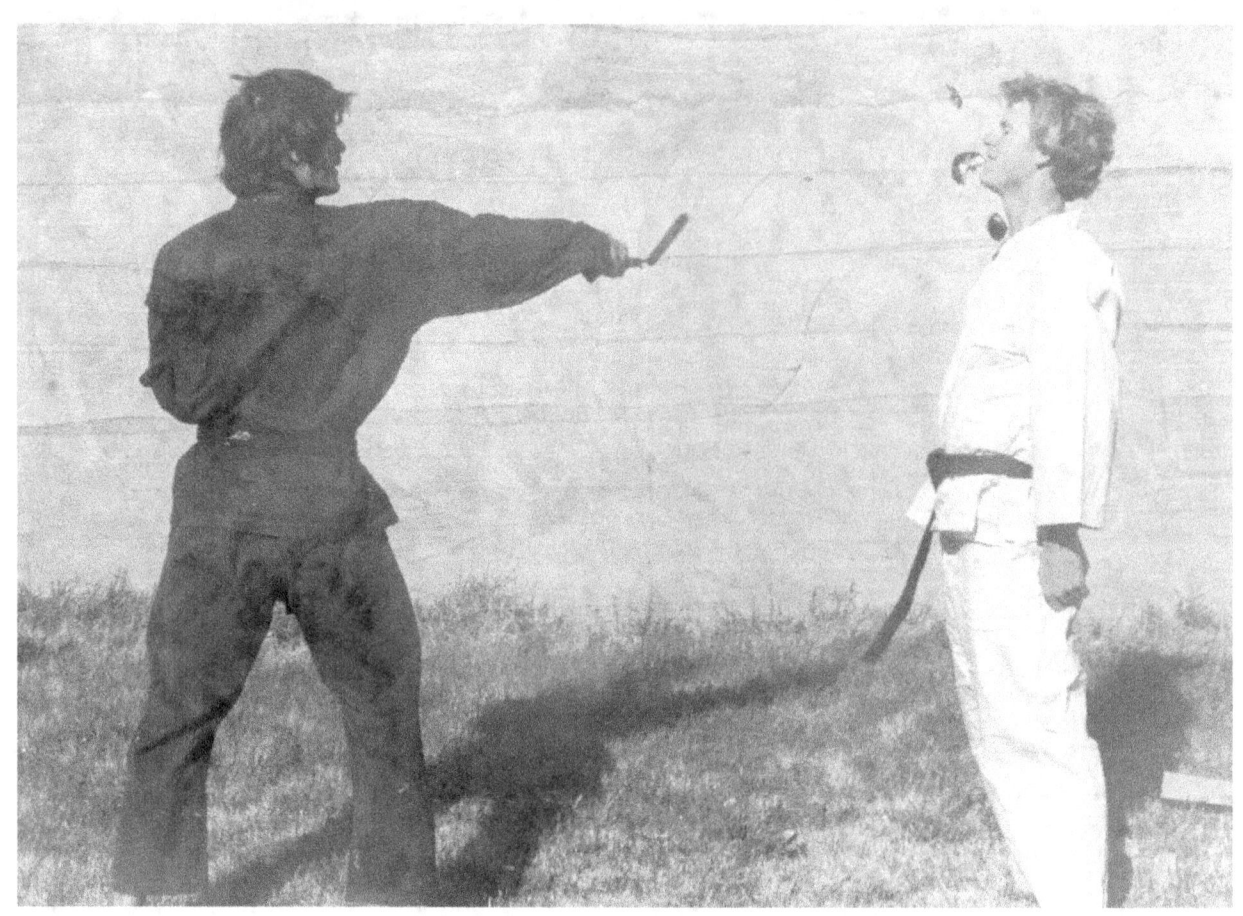

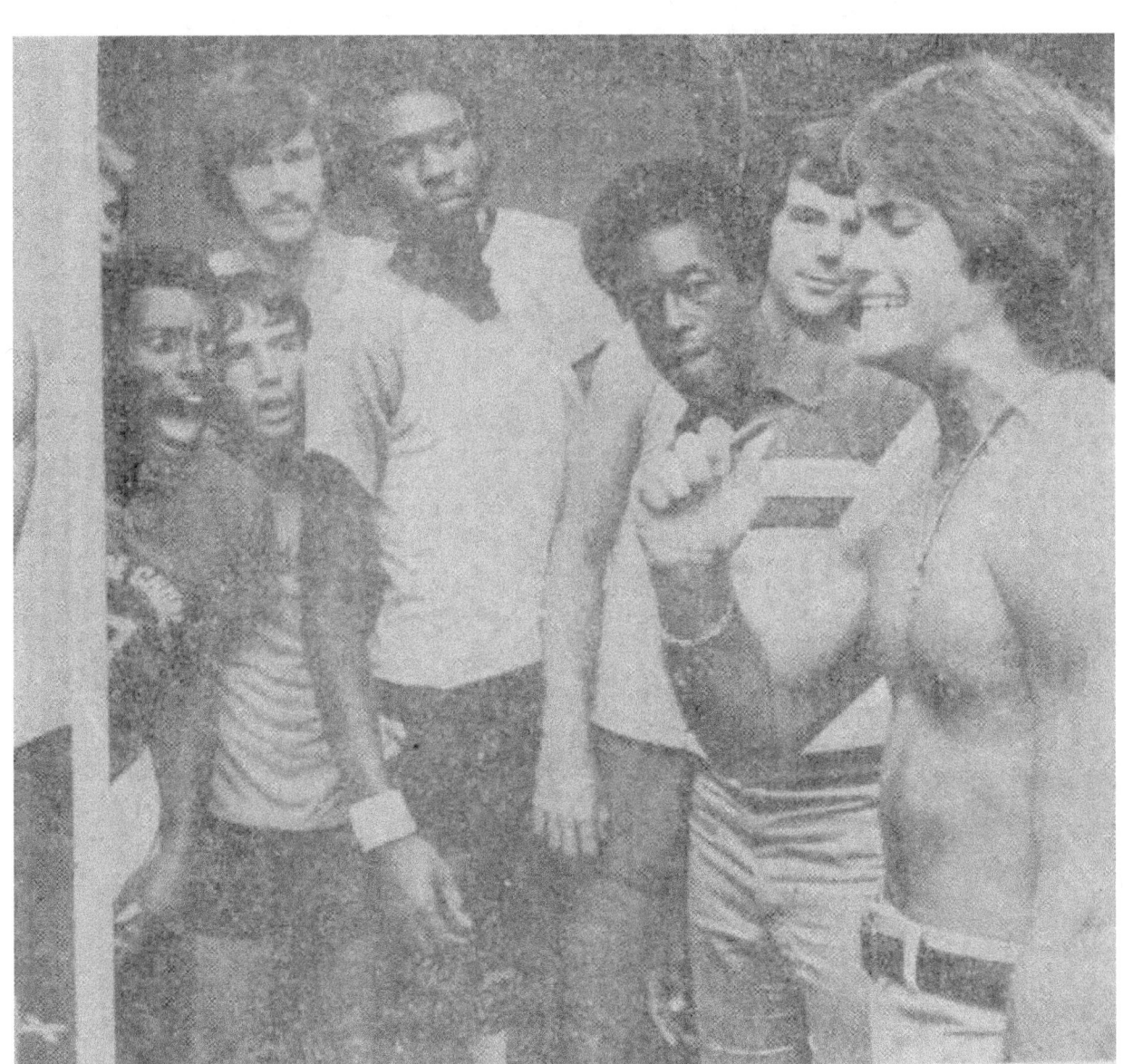

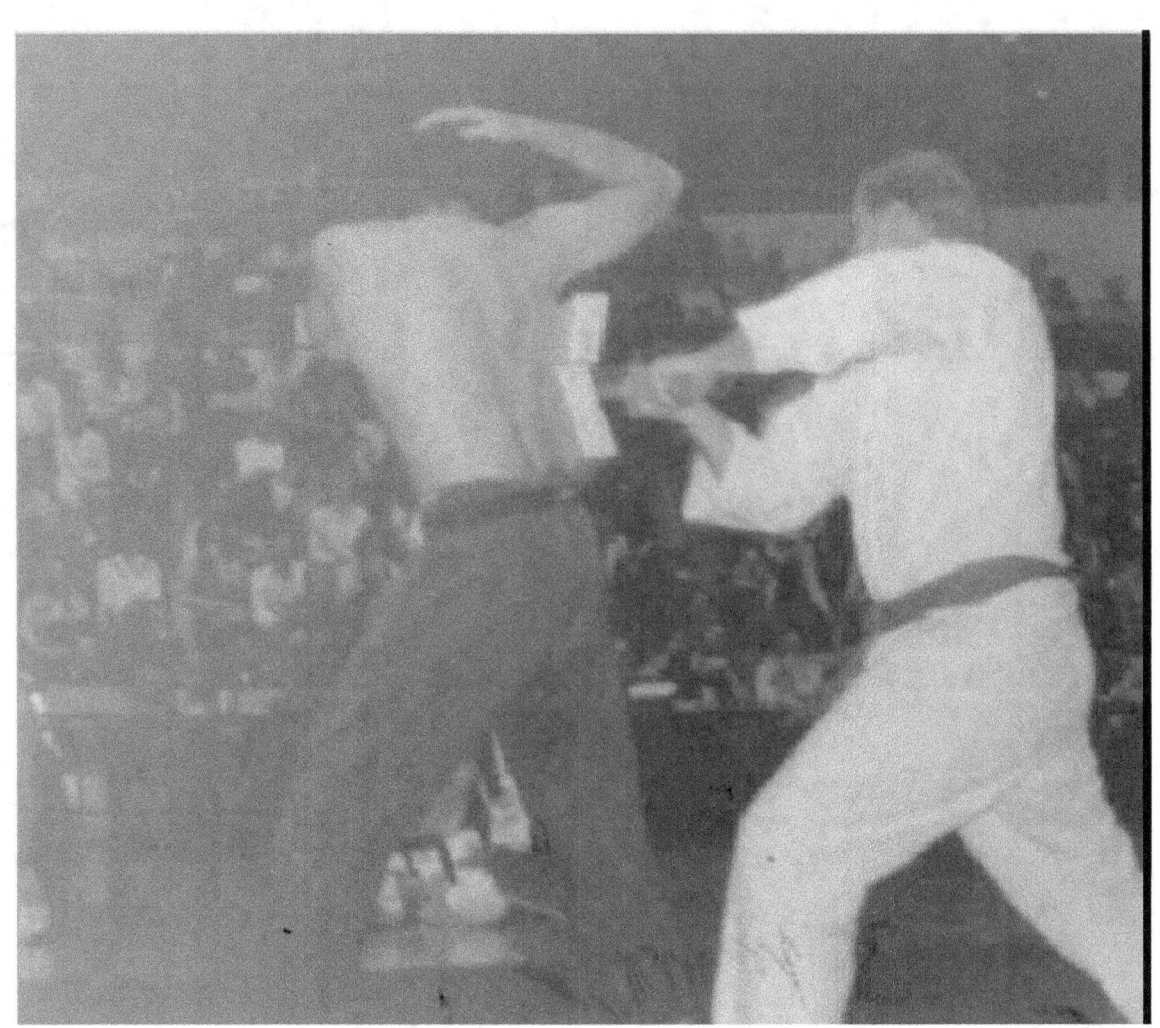

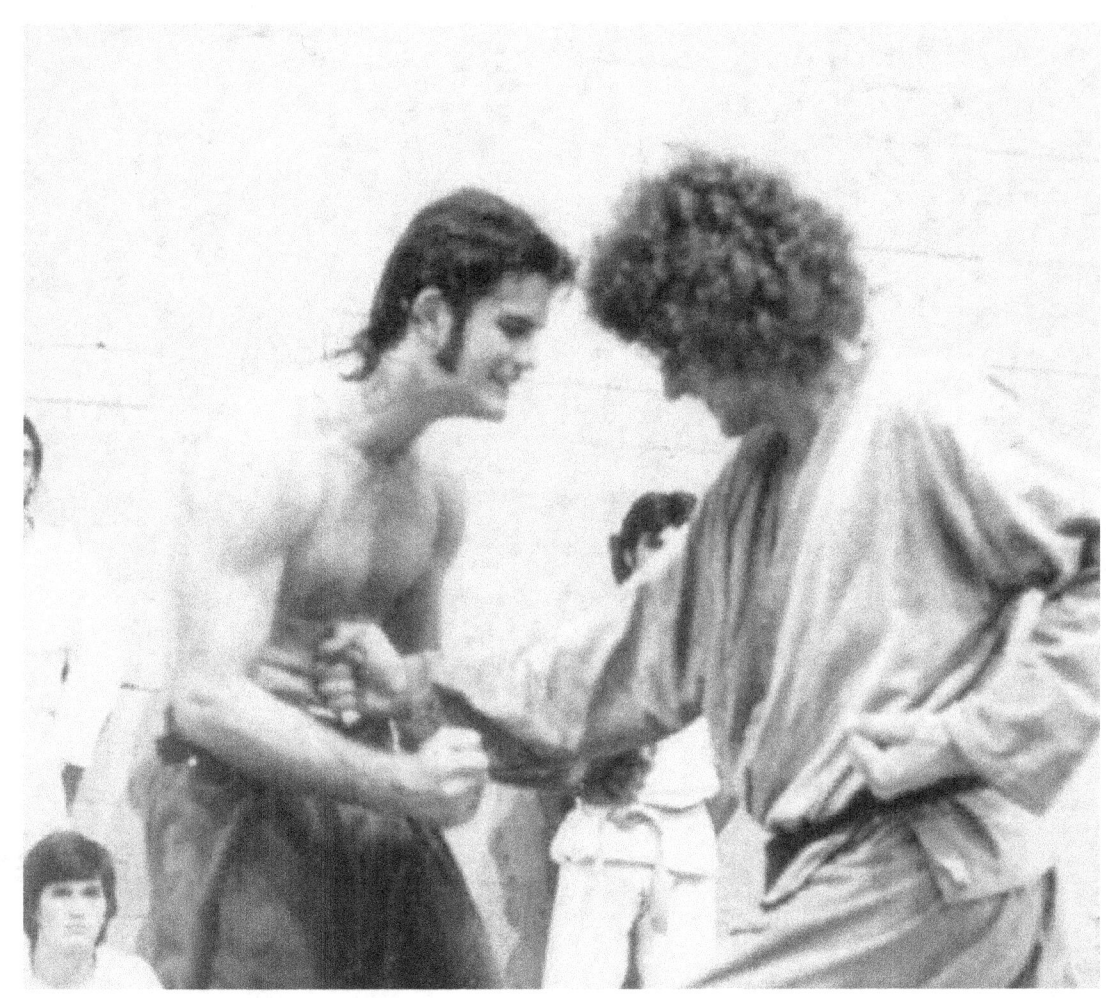

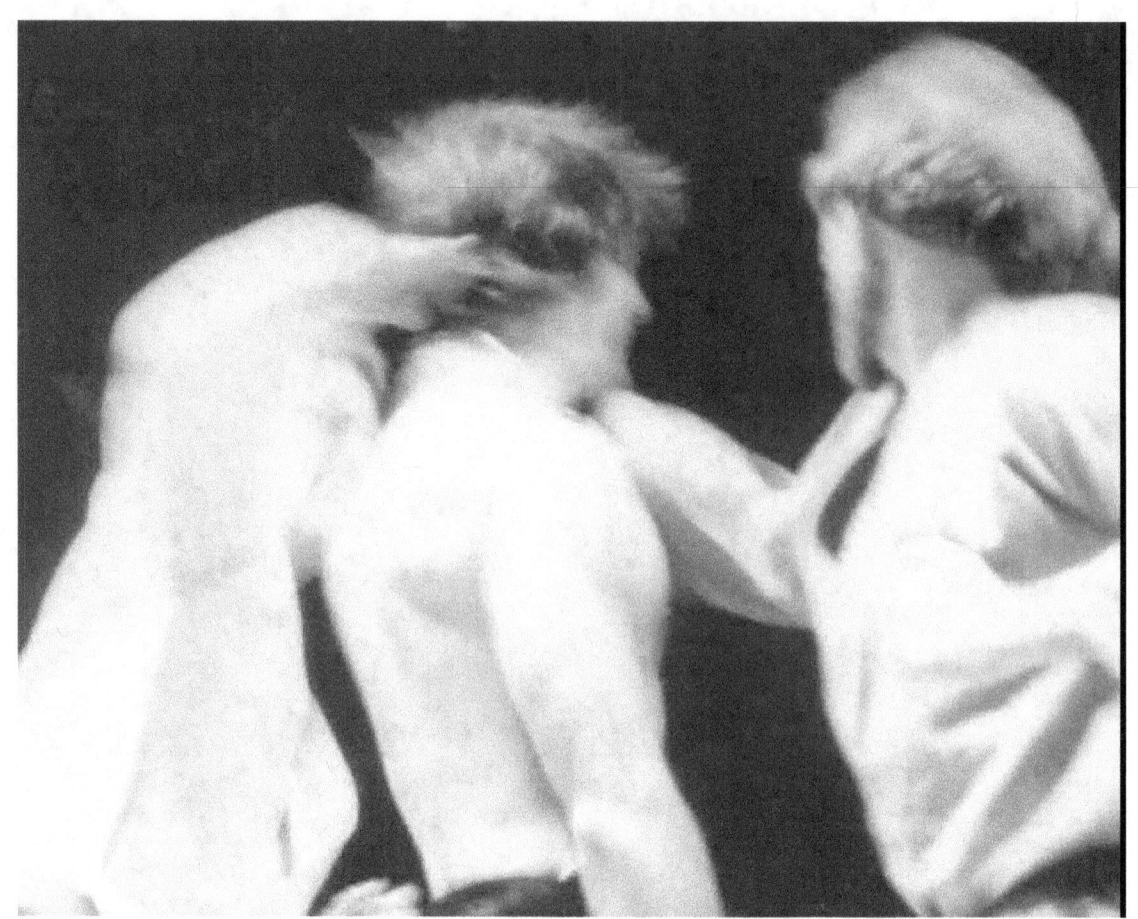

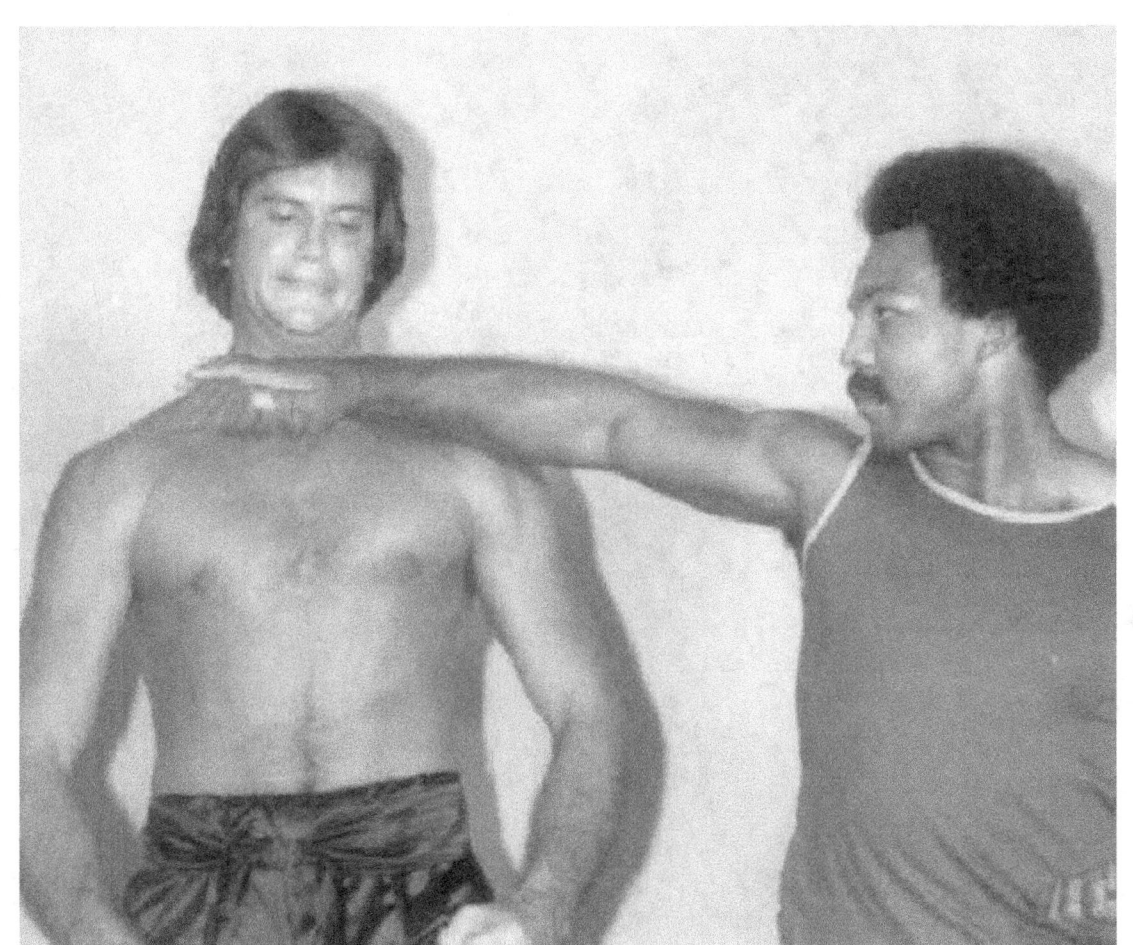

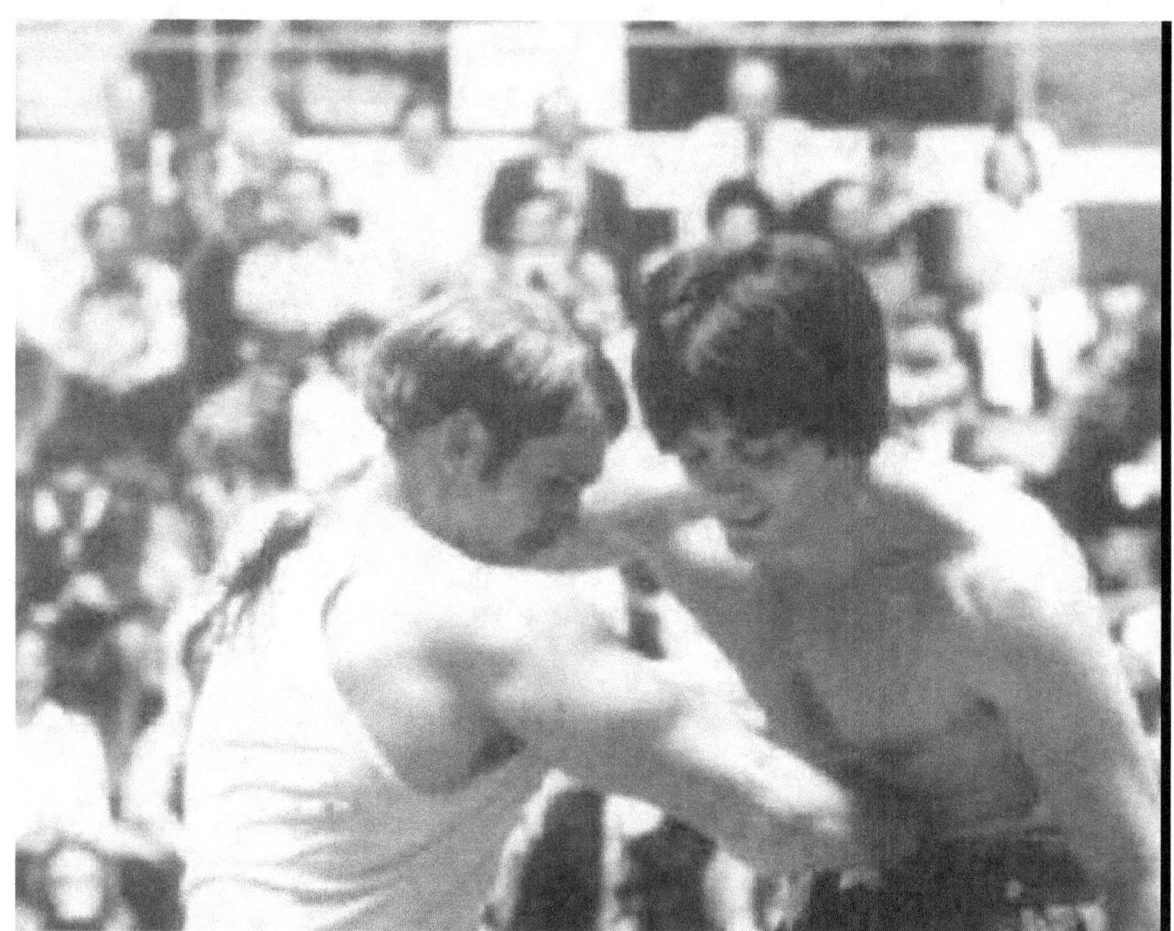

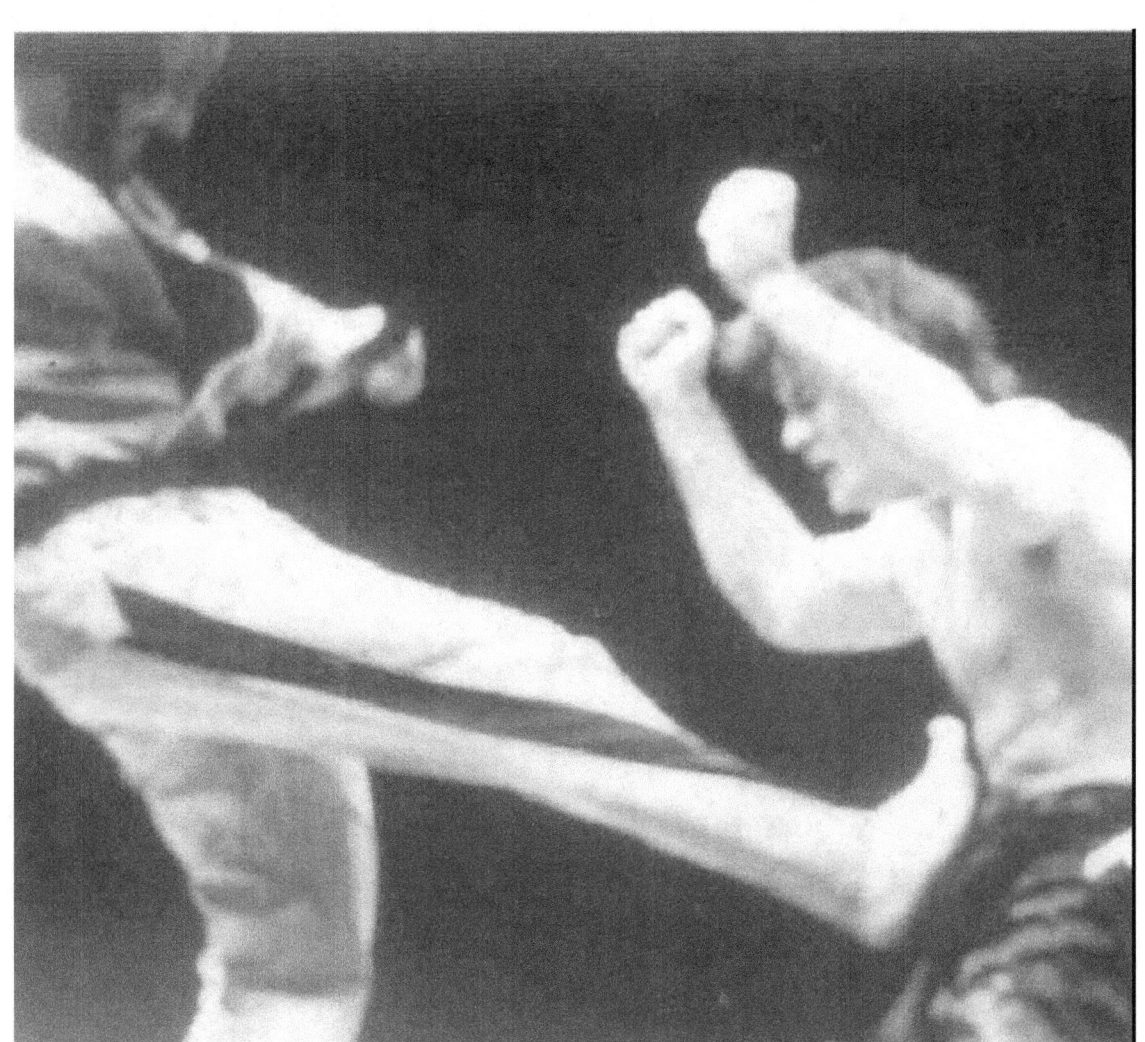

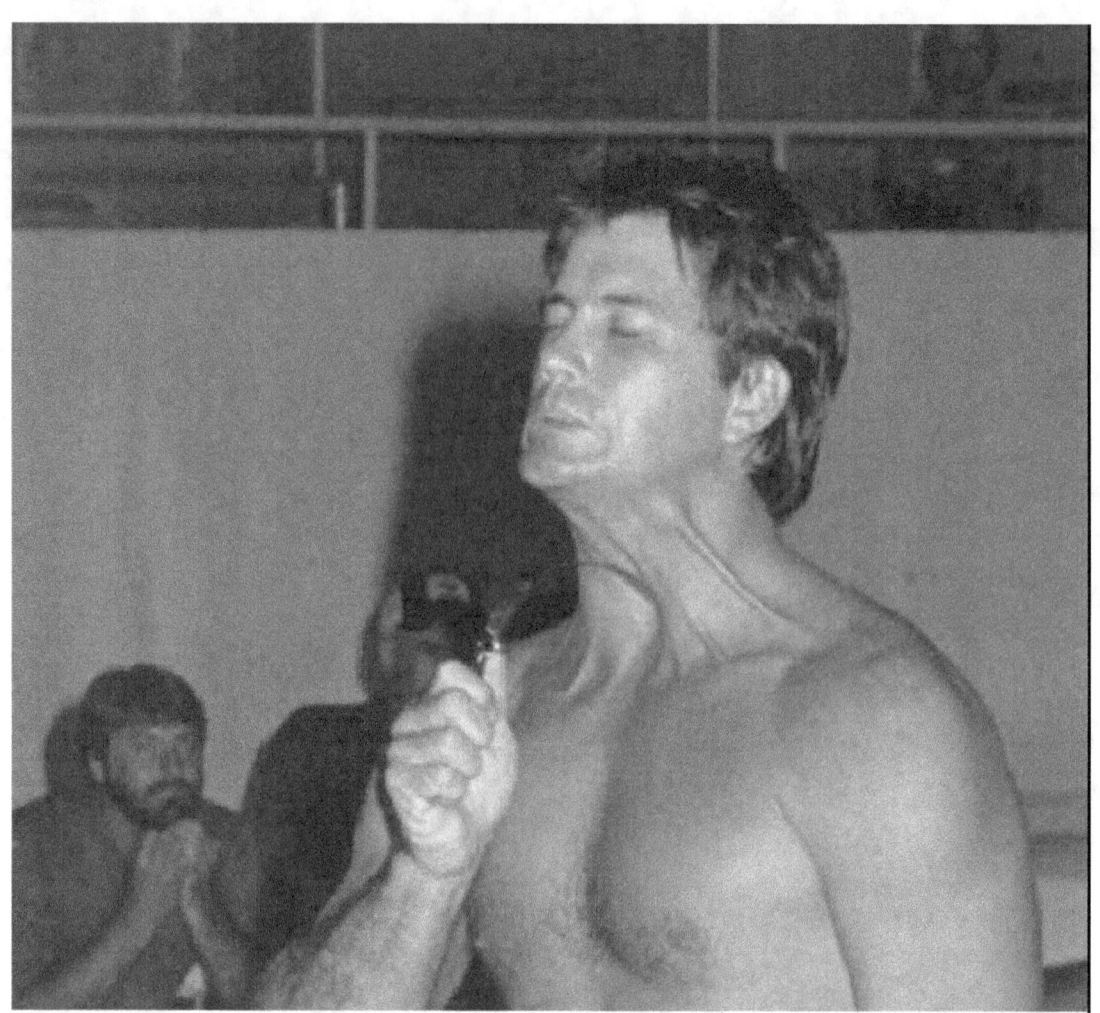

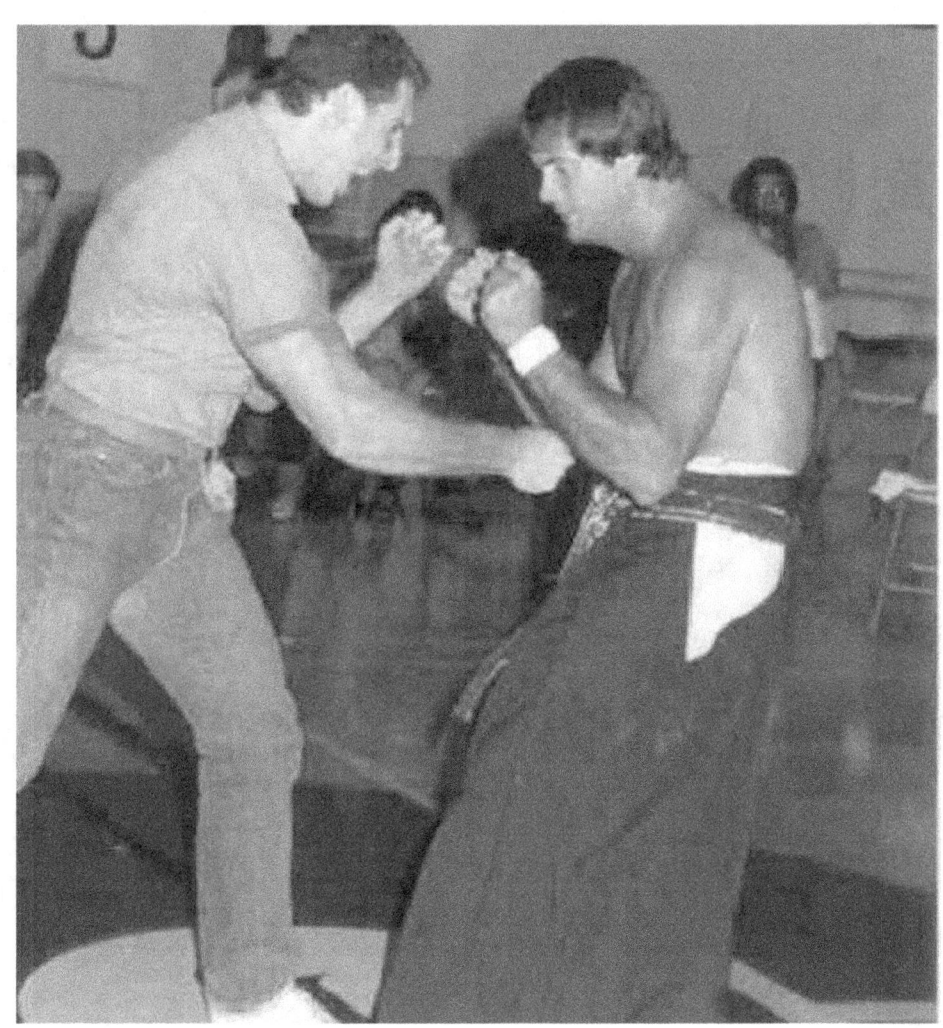

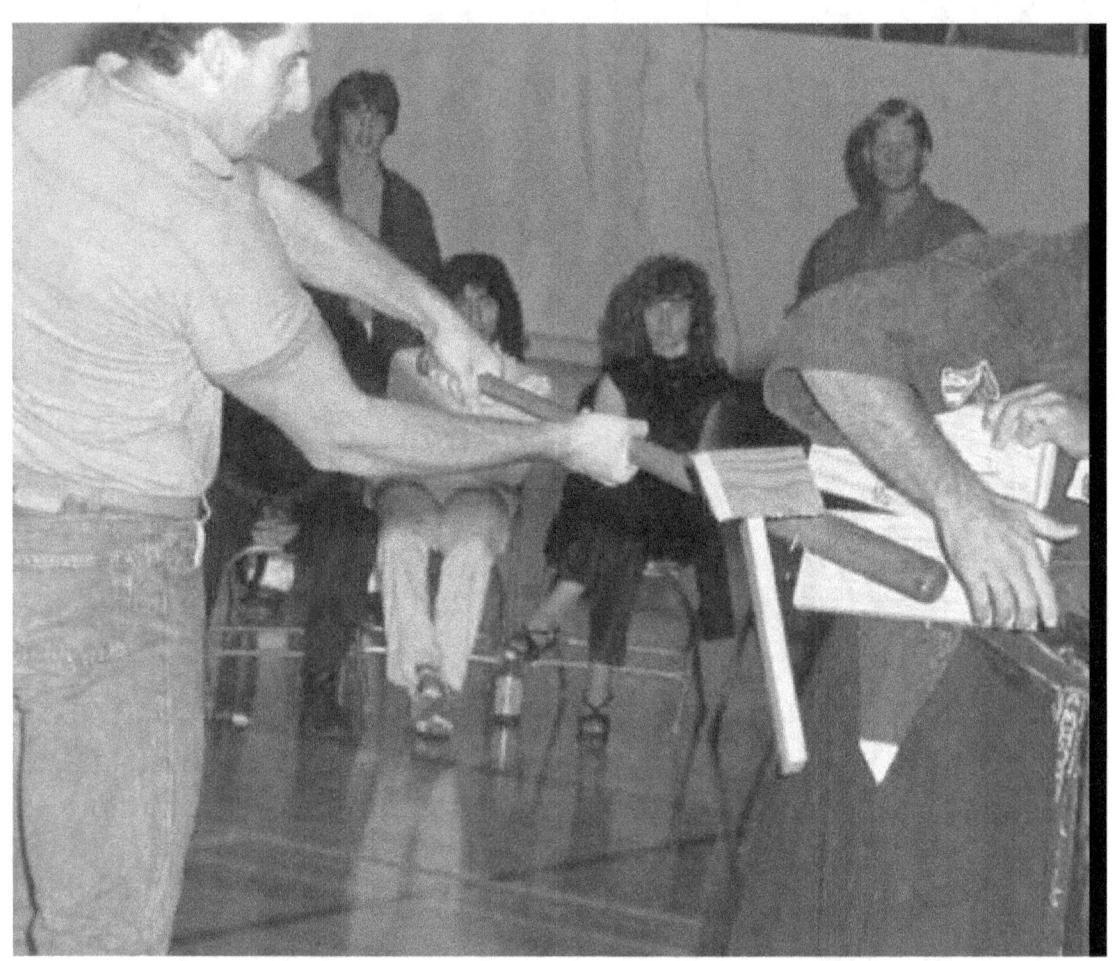